Technologic Advances and the Upper Extremity

Guest Editor

ASIF M. ILYAS, MD

HAND CLINICS

www.hand.theclinics.com

August 2010 • Volume 26 • Number 3

SAUNDERS an imprint of ELSEVIER, Inc.

W.B. SAUNDERS COMPANY
A Division of Elsevier Inc.

1600 John F. Kennedy Blvd. • Suite 1800 • Philadelphia, Pennsylvania 19103

http://www.theclinics.com

HAND CLINICS Volume 26, Number 3
August 2010 ISSN 0749-0712, ISBN-13: 978-1-4377-2454-7

Editor: Debora Dellapena

Hand Clinics (ISSN 0749-0712) is published quarterly by Elsevier Inc., 360 Park Avenue South, New York, NY 10010-1710. Months of publication are February, May, August, and November. Business and Editorial Offices: 1600 John F. Kennedy Blvd., Ste. 1800, Philadelphia, PA 19103-2899. Customer Service Office: 3251 Riverport Lane, Maryland Heights, MO 63043. Periodicals postage paid at New York, NY and at additional mailing offices. Subscription price is $316.00 per year (domestic individuals), $491.00 per year (domestic institutions), $161.00 per year (domestic students/residents), $360.00 per year (Canadian individuals), $561.00 per year (Canadian institutions), $429.00 per year (international individuals), $561.00 per year (international institutions), and $212.00 per year (international and Canadian students/residents). Foreign air speed delivery is included in all *Clinics* subscription prices. All prices are subject to change without notice. **POSTMASTER:** Send address changes to *Hand Clinics*, Elsevier Health Sciences Division, Subscription Customer Service, 3251 Riverport Lane, Maryland Heights, MO 63043. Customer Service (orders, claims, online, change of address): Elsevier Health Sciences Division, Subscription Customer Service, 3251 Riverport Lane, Maryland Heights, MO 63043. Tel: 1-800-654-2452 (U.S. and Canada); 314-447-8871 (outside U.S. and Canada). Fax: 314-447-8029. E-mail: journalscustomerservice-usa@elsevier.com (for print support); journalsonlinesupport-usa@elsevier.com (for online support).

Reprints. For copies of 100 or more of articles in this publication, please contact the Commercial Reprints Department, Elsevier Inc., 360 Park Avenue South, New York, New York 10010-1710. Tel.: 212-633-3812; Fax: 212-462-1935; E-mail: reprints@elsevier.com.

Hand Clinics is covered in *MEDLINE/PubMed (Index Medicus), Current Contents/Clinical Medicine, EMBASE/Excerpta Medica,* and *ISI/BIOMED.*

Printed and bound by CPI Group (UK) Ltd, Croydon, CR0 4YY

Transferred to Digital Print 2011

Contributors

GUEST EDITOR

ASIF M. ILYAS, MD
Hand, Upper Extremity, and Microvascular
Surgeon, Rothman Institute; Assistant
Professor of Orthopaedic Surgery, Thomas
Jefferson University Hospital, Philadelphia,
Pennsylvania

AUTHORS

JOSHUA M. ABZUG, MD
Hand Surgery Fellow, The Philadelphia Hand
Center, Department of Orthopaedic Surgery,
Thomas Jefferson University Hospital,
Philadelphia, Pennsylvania

PEDRO K. BEREDJIKLIAN, MD
Chief, Division of Hand Surgery, Associate
Professor of Orthopaedic Surgery, Rothman
Institute, Thomas Jefferson University
Hospital, Philadelphia, Pennsylvania

PHILIP E. BLAZAR, MD
Assistant Professor of Orthopedic Surgery,
Department of Orthopaedics Surgery, Brigham
and Women's Hospital, Boston,
Massachusetts

NATHAN D. BODIN, MD, MS
Resident, Department of Orthopaedic Surgery
and Sports Medicine, Temple University
Hospital, Philadelphia, Pennsylvania

DAVID J. BOZENTKA, MD
Associate Professor and Chief, Hand Surgery
Section, Department of Orthopedic Surgery,
University of Pennsylvania School
of Medicine; Chief, Department of Orthopedic
Surgery, Penn Presbyterian Medical Center,
Philadelphia, Pennsylvania

NEAL C. CHEN, MD
Clinical Lecturer, Medsport, Department of
Orthopaedic Surgery, University of Michigan,
Ann Arbor, Michigan

PHANI K. DANTULURI, MD
Assistant Professor of Orthopaedics,
Department of Orthopaedics, Emory University
Midtown Hospital; Atlanta Medical Center,
Resurgens Orthopaedics, Atlanta, Georgia

MATTHEW D. EICHENBAUM, MD
Fellow of Hand Surgery, The Philadelphia Hand
Center, Thomas Jefferson University Hospital,
Philadelphia, Pennsylvania

JOHN R. FOWLER, MD
Orthopaedic Surgery Resident, Temple
University Hospital, Philadelphia, Pennsylvania

THIERRY G. GUITTON, MSc
Research Fellow, Orthopaedic Hand and
Upper Extremity Service, Massachusetts
General Hospital, Harvard Medical School,
Boston, Massachusetts

JENNIFER HAGOPIAN, MS, ATC
Coordinator, Temple Hand Center, Temple
University Hospital, Philadelphia, Pennsylvania

KEVIN HARRELD, MD
Chief Resident, Department of Orthopaedic
Surgery, Wake Forest University School of
Medicine, Winston-Salem, North Carolina

ASIF M. ILYAS, MD
Hand, Upper Extremity, and Microvascular
Surgeon, Rothman Institute; Assistant
Professor of Orthopaedic Surgery, Thomas
Jefferson University Hospital, Philadelphia,
Pennsylvania

ROMAN ISAAC, MD
Department of Orthopaedics, New York
Medical College, St Vincent's Hospital,
New York, New York

ABHISHEK JULKA, MD
Resident Physician, Department of
Orthopaedic Surgery, University of Michigan,
Ann Arbor, Michigan

JESSE B. JUPITER, MD
Hansjorg Wyss AO Professor, Department
of Orthopaedic Surgery; Director,
Orthopaedic Hand Service, Hand and Upper
Extremity Service, Massachusetts General
Hospital, Harvard Medical School, Boston,
Massachusetts

DANTE LEVEN
Department of Orthopaedics Surgery, Brigham
and Women's Hospital, Boston,
Massachusetts

ZHONGYU LI, MD, PhD
Assistant Professor, Department of
Orthopaedic Surgery, Wake Forest University
School of Medicine, Winston-Salem,
North Carolina

JAMES T. MONICA, MD
Fellow, Hand and Upper Extremity Surgery
Service, Department of Orthopaedic Surgery,
Massachusetts General Hospital, Harvard
Medical School, Boston, Massachusetts

**CHAITANYA S. MUDGAL, MD, MS(Orth),
MCh(Orth)**
Attending Staff, Hand and Upper Extremity
Service, Massachusetts General Hospital,
Harvard Medical School; Instructor,
Department of Orthopaedic Surgery, Harvard
Medical School; Director, Hand and Upper
Extremity Surgery Fellowship, Boston,
Massachusetts

JUNG H. PARK, MD
Orthopaedic Surgery Resident, Department
of Orthopaedic Surgery, Temple University
Hospital, Philadelphia, Pennsylvania

SAQIB REHMAN, MD
Director of Orthopaedic Trauma, Temple
University Hospital; Assistant Professor,
Department of Orthopaedic Surgery; Assistant
Professor, Department of Anatomy and Cell
Biology, Temple University School of Medicine,
Philadelphia, Pennsylvania

DAVID RING, MD, PhD
Associate Professor of Orthopaedic Surgery,
Orthopaedic Hand and Upper Extremity
Service, Massachusetts General Hospital,
Harvard Medical School, Boston,
Massachusetts

MICHAEL RIVLIN, MD
Department of Orthopaedics, Thomas
Jefferson University Hospital, Philadelphia,
Pennsylvania

DAVID E. RUCHELSMAN, MD
Attending Staff, Hand and Upper Extremity
Service, Massachusetts General Hospital,
Harvard Medical School; Instructor,
Department of Orthopaedic Surgery, Harvard
Medical School, Boston, Massachusetts

GBOLABO SOKUNBI, MD
Department of Orthopaedic Surgery, Temple
University Hospital, Philadelphia, Pennsylvania

EMRAN SHEIKH, MD
Division of Hand Surgery, Rothman Institute,
Thomas Jefferson University Hospital,
Philadelphia, Pennsylvania

EON K. SHIN, MD
Assistant Professor of Orthopedic Surgery,
The Philadelphia Hand Center, Thomas
Jefferson University Hospital, Philadelphia,
Pennsylvania

RYAN SPANGLER, BS
Temple University School of Medicine,
Philadelphia, Pennsylvania

JOSEPH J. THODER, MD, FACS
Professor and Chairman, Department
of Orthopaedic Surgery and Sports Medicine,
Temple University Hospital, Philadelphia,
Pennsylvania

Contents

> Locked fixed-angle plating in the hand and wrist helps to optimize outcomes following surgical fixation of select acute fractures and complex reconstructions. Select indications include unstable distal ulna head/neck fractures, periarticular metacarpal and phalangeal fractures, comminuted/multifragmentary diaphyseal fractures with bone loss (ie, combined injuries of the hand), osteopenic/pathologic fractures, nonunions and corrective osteotomy fixation, and small joint arthrodesis. Locked plating techniques in the hand should not be seen as a panacea for wrist and digital acute trauma and delayed reconstructions. An understanding of the biomechanics of fixed-angle plating and proper technical application of locking constructs will optimize outcomes and minimize complications. As clinical experience with locking technology in hand trauma broadens, new indications and applications will emerge. Currently, several systems are available. The specific implants share common features in their protocols for insertion, but unique differences in their design (ie, individual locking mechanisms, uniaxial vs polyaxial locking capability, metallurgy, and plate profiles) must be appreciated and considered preoperatively.

> Metacarpal fractures are common, especially in men, and account for about 10% of all fractures in patients. The fracture pattern and location, and the degree of angulation are important in determining the optimal treatment approach. Although metacarpal fractures can be treated nonsurgically, certain indications such as irreducible fractures, malrotations, and open fractures may necessitate surgery. Intramedullary nail fixation has been successful in treating metacarpal fractures. Complications can be minimized by taking appropriate precautions and care in performing the surgery.

> Resection arthroplasty with or without ligament reconstruction for thumb trapeziometacarpal arthritis can be complicated by thumb shortening and pinch-strength weakness. Implant arthroplasties have been developed to limit loss of thumb length, improve strength, and limit postoperative convalescence. The ideal thumb carpometacarpal implant should be strong and stable, provide full range of motion, and prevent loosening. Unfortunately, no current prosthesis accomplishes all of these goals. Until the ideal implant is developed, clinical acumen must be used to determine appropriate patients and implants.

> Carpometacarpal (CMC) arthritis of the thumb affects half of postmenopausal women and up to 25% of elderly men. This disease can cause significant disability

in affected patients often necessitating surgical intervention. Various surgical options have been used to treat refractory CMC arthritis. Any successful surgical intervention must address three goals: removal of diseased joint surfaces, reconstruction of ligamentous stabilizers, and preservation of the joint space. In this article we will discuss various interposition arthroplasty options for CMC arthritis of the thumb.

Scaphoid fractures carry significant long-term morbidity and short-term socioeconomic difficulty in the young and active patient population in which they most commonly occur. While cast immobilization results in high rates of radiographic union in nondisplaced scaphoid fractures, internal fixation with headless compression screws has been recommended in cases of displaced fractures. Internal fixation has led to high rates of union in both nondisplaced and displaced fractures with the added benefits of earlier mobilization and return to work and sports. Multiple manufacturers are now offering "second generation" headless compression screws for the internal fixation of scaphoid fractures. The few biomechanical studies that exist demonstrate improved compression forces and load to failure for the newer generation of headless compression screws when compared with the first generation headless compression screw, although it is unclear if these differences are clinically significant.

Intramedullary fixation is the latest in a variety of techniques that have been developed to manage distal radius fractures. Intramedullary nailing of these fractures combines the soft-tissue advantages of a less invasive surgical approach with the biomechanical advantages of locking screw technology. These features may enable an accelerated postoperative rehabilitation and quicker return to function. Disadvantages associated with the intramedullary technique include the necessity of a closed or percutaneous reduction and the inability of the implant to adequately stabilize intraarticular or highly comminuted fractures. Consequently, intramedullary implants are primarily indicated for fixation of extra-articular or simple intraarticular split patterns and should not be employed for management of volar or dorsal shear fractures. Preliminary clinical data is emerging in the form of short-term follow-up studies with limited numbers of study participants.

Surgical treatment options for distal radius fractures are many and commonly involve volar locked plating. More recently, newer volar locking plates have been introduced to the market that allow the placement of independent distal subchondral variable-angle locking screws to better achieve targeted fracture fixation. This article reviews this new technology and presents the authors' experience with the Aptus (Medartis, Kennett Square, Pennsylvania) variable-angle volar locking plates.

Surgical management of distal radius fractures continues to evolve because of their high incidence in an increasingly active elderly population. Traditional radiocarpal external fixation relies on ligamentotaxis for fracture reduction but has several drawbacks. Nonbridging external fixation has evolved to provide early wrist mobility in the setting of anatomic fracture reduction. Several studies of the nonbridging technique have demonstrated satisfactory results in isolated nonbridging external fixation series and in comparison with traditional spanning external fixation. Nonbridging external fixation for surgical treatment of distal radius fractures can be technically demanding and requires at least 1 cm of intact volar cortex in the distal fracture fragment for successful implementation.

Intramedullary Fixation of Forearm Fractures   391

Saqib Rehman and Gbolabo Sokunbi

Plate fixation remains the primary surgical treatment option for most adult forearm fractures. However, intramedullary nailing can be successful and might be preferable in cases of massive soft-tissue injury and burns, certain segmental fractures, pathologic fractures, and skeletally immature adolescent patients. Furthermore, the risk for refracture after plate removal is decreased with fixation by intramedullary nailing. The history, indications, surgical technique, and results of intramedullary fixation of forearm fractures are described in this article.

Radial Head Arthroplasty   403

James T. Monica and Chaitanya S. Mudgal

Radial head arthroplasty remains an encouraging treatment option for comminuted radial head fractures in an unstable elbow or forearm. This article discusses the surgical considerations related to radial head arthroplasty, including anatomy, indications, and surgical technique. Radial head arthroplasty outcomes literature and a review of current implant options are also discussed.

Use of Orthogonal or Parallel Plating Techniques to Treat Distal Humerus Fractures   411

Joshua M. Abzug and Phani K. Dantuluri

Distal humerus fractures continue to be a complex fracture to treat. This article describes two surgical techniques that can be used to tackle these difficult fractures: Parallel plating and orthogonal plating. Both techniques have yielded excellent outcomes after open reduction and internal fixation; yet each has its own set of unique considerations. However, the key to successful treatment of these difficult fractures regardless of technique remains obtaining anatomic reduction with stable fixation and the implementation of early motion.

Hinged External Fixation of the Elbow   423

Neal C. Chen and Abhishek Julka

Hinged external fixation of the elbow provides the advantages of static fixation with the benefits of continued motion through the joint. Indications for the use of this method of fixation include traumatic instability, distraction interposition arthroplasty, instability after contracture release, and instability after excision of heterotopic ossification. Orthopedic surgeons should be familiar with hinged fixators and their application when faced with an unstable ulnohumeral joint.

Hand Clinics

THE CLINICS ARE NOW AVAILABLE ONLINE!

Access your subscription at:
www.theclinics.com

Preface

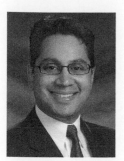

Asif M. Ilyas, MD
Guest Editor

We are living in a period of rapid technological advances in the field of medicine. Nowhere are these advances more obvious that in the subspecialties of orthopaedic surgery, particularly in hand and upper extremity surgery. These new tools and techniques have resulted in a spectrum of changes to the way we manage our practice and approach upper extremity pathologies. Examples of these advances include locking plates for fractures of the hand and wrist, new-generation headless compression screws, new intramedullary nailing techniques, new metal and soft tissue arthroplasty options for the basal joint of the thumb, varied elbow fracture treatment approaches, and increased nerve repair options. In some cases these advances have augmented our traditional treatment modalities and in other cases they have completely revolutionized our treatment paradigm.

To most optimally apply these new tools, a thorough understanding of their features and limitations is necessary. Optimal outcomes require diligent technique and appropriate indications. In this issue, the chapter authors and I review in detail some of the more pivotal upper extremity technologic advances and attempt to provide the reader with best evidence guidelines for their application.

Asif M. Ilyas, MD
Rothman Institute
Thomas Jefferson University Hospital
925 Chestnut Street
Philadelphia, PA 19107, USA

E-mail address:
aimd2001@yahoo.com

doi:10.1016/j.hcl.2010.05.012

hand.theclinics.com

The Role of Locking Technology in the Hand

David E. Ruchelsman, MD[a,b],
Chaitanya S. Mudgal, MD, MS(Orth), MCh(Orth)[a,b,c],
Jesse B. Jupiter, MD[a,b,*]

KEYWORDS

- Locking plates • Metacarpal and phalanx fractures
- Hand trauma

Internal fixation of the hand and wrist has evolved in the last 4 decades. It is well accepted that stable internal fixation in the setting of combined musculoskeletal injuries involving the osseous skeleton and soft-tissue envelope facilitates early rehabilitation and promotes improved functional outcomes.[1–4] Plate and screw fixation systems in the hand and wrist were originally predicated on the larger long-bone fracture fixation systems. Locked plating establishes a fixed-angle construct (ie, functions as an internal-external fixator). Angular-stable fixation has begun to revolutionize the operative management of complex metadiaphyseal long-bone trauma, as well as periarticular and periprosthetic fractures, and has acquired a growing role in the hand as well.

With the growth of hand surgery as a subspecialty, and a better understanding of the structural requirements of the hand skeleton and periarticular soft tissues, an increasing number of commercially available hand fracture fixation systems that incorporate fixed-angle technology into plate and screw designs have emerged. The multiple hand fracture locking plate systems available reflect the growing trend amongst hand surgeons to use internal fixation for difficult acute fractures (ie,

acute bone loss, periarticular and metaphyseal fractures, osteopenic bone) and complex reconstructions for malunion, nonunion, or posttraumatic deformities. Locked plates in the hand confer rigid or relative stability based on the clinical scenario being addressed.

In appropriately selected cases, locking plate technology may be helpful in addressing a variety of extraarticular and periarticular problems in the hand and wrist. Clinical experience with locking technology in hand trauma remains relatively limited compared with its application for fractures about the proximal humerus,[5–8] distal humerus,[9] distal radius,[10–14] distal femur,[15,16] periprosthetic femur,[17,18] tibial plateau,[19] proximal,[20] and distal tibia.[21] As hand surgeons become more familiar with locked plating, these plates may augment or replace the use of the technically demanding fixed-angle blade plates used to stabilize periarticular fractures and osteotomies.

The current indications and impetus for locked (fixed-angle) plating, along with the pearls and pitfalls of this technology are highlighted by anatomic region in the hand. Results following the application of locking plate technology in the management of distal radius acute fractures[10–14]

[a] Hand and Upper Extremity Service, Yawkey Center, Massachusetts General Hospital, Harvard Medical School, 55 Fruit Street, Suite 2100, MA 02114, USA
[b] Department of Orthopaedic Surgery, Harvard Medical School, Boston, 55 Fruit Street, Suite 2100, MA 02114, USA
[c] Hand and Upper Extremity Surgery Fellowship, Harvard Medical School, 55 Fruit Street, Suite 2100, Boston, MA 02114, USA
* Corresponding author. Hand and Upper Extremity Service, Yawkey Center, Massachusetts General Hospital, Harvard Medical School, 55 Fruit Street, Suite 2100, Boston, MA 02114.
E-mail address: jjupiter1@partners.org

Hand Clin 26 (2010) 307–319
doi:10.1016/j.hcl.2010.04.001

and malunion[22,23] have been extensively reported. A discussion of locked plating in the distal radius is beyond the scope of this article. The application of locking technology in the distal ulna, metacarpals, and phalanges is discussed here.

BIOMECHANICS
Conventional Compression Plating

Conventional nonlocked plate/screw constructs rely on frictional force created between the plate and bone surface to neutralize the axial, torsional, and 3-point bending forces experienced by the plate/screw/bone construct.[24] Stability with standard plate/screw constructs is largely determined by screw torque generated. Osteopenia, metaphyseal bone, comminution, segmental bone loss, and/or pathologic bone all affect maximal screw-thread purchase and compromise the development of sufficient torque to establish absolute stability with compression plating.[24,25] However, the need to perform a more extensive soft-tissue dissection to maximize the plate-bone contact interface and coefficient of friction with conventional plating systems may adversely affect the fracture site and periosteal biology.

Locked Fixed-Angle Plating

Early attempts at improving fixation of conventional plates to compromised bone have included the use of bone cement to improve screw torque, Schuhli nuts,[26] and Zespol plates[27] to create a fixed-angle construct. Fixed-angle technology has been refined by the Arbeitsgemeinschaft fur Osteosynthesefragen (AO/ASIF) group.[28-32] In the Synthes (Paoli, PA, USA) fracture fixation system, the locking screw heads are conical with threads that lock into corresponding screw hole threads that are recessed within the body of the plate. A recent proliferation of locked plate designs by several manufacturers has followed. Locking technology aims to eliminate screw toggle and to create a fixed-angle single-beam construct.[33] Endosteal fibula allograft augmentation[34] has been described as a supplemental technique to locked plating in larger long bones.

Locked fixed-angle plate/screw constructs function as an internal-external fixator. Locked plates preserve periosteal vascularity while maintaining fixation by locking the fixation screws to the plate, which may be placed extraperiosteally. The angular stability of locked screws functions to distribute the applied load more evenly across the component screws, thus avoiding significant load concentration at a single screw-bone interface.[24,35,36] In a locked plate system, the overall strength equals the sum of fixation strengths of all screw-bone interfaces instead of that of a single component screw as in conventional plating. As a result, the fixed-angle construct leads to a mechanism of screw-purchase failure that is fundamentally different from that of conventional unlocked screws. Locked screws act together in parallel, whereas conventional screws act in series.[35] With 3-point bending load application, screw hole track deformation occurs. Unlocked screws toggle within the screw track and sequentially loosen. In contrast, with fixed-angle fixation, the plate/screw construct must fail as a unit.

Locked plates may be used in a bridging mode across an area of comminution and/or bone loss, thereby avoiding fracture site compression. Bridge plating helps to preserve the vascularity of the intercalary fracture fragments. Relative stability is achieved and allows enough strain at the fracture site to promote secondary bone healing with callus formation.[37] Alternatively, locked screws can be used to augment a standard compression plate/screw construct to create hybrid fixation (ie, non-locked and locked screws). In a hybrid construct, it is therefore essential to apply compression across the fracture site using standard techniques before insertion of the locked screws. The use of hybrid fixation with bicortical locking screws is advantageous in osteopenic bone.

Indeed, current locked plate designs incorporate combination-hole technology, which allows surgeons to incorporate aspects of locked plating and compression plating into a single implant and at each screw hole site. Combination plates are helpful in select fracture patterns in which one aspect of the fracture would benefit from anatomic reduction and compression (ie, simple intraarticular component), whereas another fracture component would benefit from bridging fixation (ie, comminuted metadiaphyseal portion). If cortical contact can be achieved on the compression side, it is essential to complete maximal fracture compression before locked screws are inserted.

INDICATIONS

Current indications for locked plating in the hand include unstable distal ulna head/neck fractures associated with unstable fracture of the distal radius, periarticular metacarpal and phalangeal fractures, especially those with metaphyseal comminution, complex multifragmentary diaphyseal fractures with bone loss (ie, open, combined injuries of the hand), osteopenic/pathologic fractures, fixation for nonunions and corrective osteotomies in the hand, and arthrodeses of the small joints of the hand.

CONTRAINDICATIONS

There are no absolute contraindications to the use of locked plates in the hand and wrist. However, there are scenarios for which fixed-angle locked plating is not essential. If open reduction internal fixation is selected for simple, displaced, diaphyseal fractures of the short tubular bones in nonosteopenic patients, compression or neutralization with nonlocking plate fixation is all that is required. In addition, simple intraarticular split fractures do not require locked plating. With increasing emphasis on cost-effectiveness in the practice of medicine, the added cost associated with locking plates remains a concern.[38] We believe that locked fixation in the hand should be reserved for problematic fractures that are expected to have suboptimal outcomes using conventional plate/screw constructs.

Percutaneous insertion of fixed-angle plates is now performed routinely for distal femur, proximal and distal tibia, and pediatric diaphyseal fractures while adhering to AO principles of internal fixation. Cited advantages include percutaneous reduction, extraperiosteal plate placement, and bridging fixation. In the hand and wrist, the intricate association of the flexor and extensor tendons and neurovascular structures to the bones prohibit percutaneous insertion of percutaneous plate/screw constructs.

CONTEMPORARY ANGULAR-STABLE DESIGNS

Fixed-angle implants were introduced more than 20 years ago by Buchler and Fisher.[39] These investigators reported their initial experience with the minicondylar plate (Synthes, Paoli, PA, USA) for periarticular metacarpal and phalangeal fractures. The design of this fixed-angle implant was predicated on larger blade plates used extensively for periarticular fractures in other anatomic locations (ie, proximal and distal femur) (**Fig. 1**). The minicondylar plate was initially made of steel and available in 1.5-mm and 2.0-mm sizes. It is currently also available in titanium. Blade length is determined by predrilling the blade pathway. The blade is then inserted and acts as a derotation device and resists shear on the condylar fragments. Condylar fracture fragments can also be fixed and compressed with the supplemental condylar screw.

Proper insertion of this device remains technically challenging.[3,40] The evolution of small locking plates for hand applications may minimize the complications reported with minicondylar plates. Fixed-angle locking subarticular buttress pins are an alternative to the use of the minicondylar blade plate.

Novel plate/screw locking mechanisms continue to emerge. These advances have recently led to the introduction of polyaxial locking capabilities in addition to fixed monoaxial locking designs. Multiple factors are responsible for the proliferation of new locked plate designs by several manufacturers. These include improved biomaterials, the desire for anatomically precontoured plates, and the need to respect company-specific patents. Biomechanical analyses in cadaveric specimens have previously validated the use of these low-profile plates.[41–43] Studies reporting clinical and radiographic outcomes following dedicated use of the current systems are needed to further define their applications.

Synthes

The AO/ASIF group (Synthes, Paoli, PA, USA) has developed the minifragment and modular hand locking compression plate (LCP) fixation systems. Both modules are available in 316L stainless steel and titanium alloy. Self-tapping cortical and locking screws are available in the 2.7-mm, 2.4-mm, and 2.0-mm minifragment and modular hand trays.

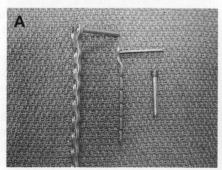 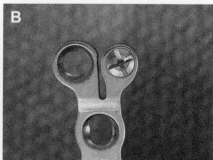

Fig. 1. Contemporary minicondylar locking plate (*right*) and blade plate (*middle*) (Synthes, Paoli, PA). The subarticular locking buttress screws have threaded heads (*left*) (*A*) which lock into the screw hole, creating a fixed-angle construct (*B*).

The LCP plates are unique in that they offer sequential combi-holes that afford either cortical or locking screw fixation through the same hole (**Fig. 2**). In this system, the locking screw heads are conical with threads that lock into the screw hole threads. The locking screw angle is monoaxial, and is dictated by the trajectory of the locking sleeve insert into the locking side of the combi-hole. The 2.4-mm condylar plate uses a 1.8-mm locking subarticular buttress pin. Additional nonlocking 1.5-mm and 1.3-mm plates are found in the modular hand fracture fixation system. Plates are available in straight, Y-, T-, and H-shaped configurations . Notched plates facilitate plate cutting and additional contouring. These low-profile plates (plate thickness range, 0.7–1.25 mm)[44] make periosteal closure around the implant easier.

Stryker

The Stryker VariAx Hand Locking Module (Stryker-Leibinger, Kalamazoo, MI, USA) builds on this company's Profyle Hand Standard Plating Module,[44] a nonlocking plate/screw system with 2.3-mm, 1.7-mm, and 1.2-mm implant options. The VariAx module offers polyaxial locking plate/screws in 2.3 mm and 1.7 mm (maximum plate thickness, 1.5 mm). Anatomically precontoured plates in variable shapes and lengths provide multiple fixation options in each region of the hand (**Fig. 3**). An oblong shaft hole allows proper positioning relative to the periarticular segment head and collateral ligament recesses.

This system offers polyaxial (ie, variable angle) locking interfaces. The lip on the drill guide allows for toggle within a 20° arc (±10° in each direction) when it engages the screw hole. Every angle in this angular cone results in locking of the screw. Polyaxial locking allows the surgeon to dictate the precise placement of the locking screws based on plate positioning, fracture characteristics, and proximity to the articular surface. Their locking mechanism is created as the stronger grade 5 titanium alloy in the screw head obtains purchase within the screw hole made of softer grade 2

titanium in these plates. The locking threads on the underside of the screw head also engage the circular lip in the screw hole. Rounded low-profile screw heads minimize soft-tissue irritation when the locking screw is inserted at the maximum allowable angle. Similar to the Synthes fixation system, all plate holes (with the exception of the oblong shaft screw holes) can be filled with either nonlocking or locking screws, and thus allows for creation of a hybrid fixation construct. As opposed to combi-holes, each hole is circular, and locking is created by use of a locking screw made of grade 5 titanium alloy. In osteopenic bone, locked screws can be inserted to augment standard nonlocking compression screws made of grade 2 titanium. Bicortical screws are used for improved torsional control, but unicortical locking screws can also be used to avoid screw tip prominence and irritation of tendons or periarticular structures.

Medartis

The Medartis (Basel, Switzerland) Aptus titanium system offers 2.0-mm and 2.3-mm plate and screw options for angular-stable fixation of metacarpal and phalangeal fractures (plate thicknesses,1.0 mm and 1.3 mm, respectively). Screw holes are offset to reduce screw collision and are also oriented in a nonlinear configuration to avoid fracture propagation with drilling. Locking is achieved through a TriLock radial 3-point wedge-locking mechanism (**Fig. 4**). TriLock locking screws can be re-locked in the same hole under individual angles up to 3 times. This system also offers polyaxial locking capabilities within a 15° cone. The 1.2-mm and 1.5-mm phalangeal plates do not offer a locking option.

DePuy

DePuy (Warsaw, IN, USA) has recently introduced its 1.5-mm and 2.5-mm titanium ALPS for hand reconstruction (plate thicknesses, 1.1 mm and 1.6 mm, respectively). Plate styles include straight, T, Y, web, and T/Y options (**Fig. 5**). Nonlocking as well as monoaxial and polyaxial locking interfaces are available at each screw hole in the 1.5-mm and 2.5-mm plates. Preloaded fixed-angle screw targeting (FAST) guides facilitate rapid insertion of nonlocking cortical screws and monoaxial locking screws. 2.5-mm and 1.5-mm polyaxial (20° locking cone; ±10° in each direction off center) locking screws are also available and are predrilled after removing the FAST guides. These multidirectional locking screws are made of cobalt-chrome and the threaded screw heads create a new thread path in the plate (see **Fig. 5**). In addition, 1.5-mm nonlocking screws placed eccentrically or 2.5-mm

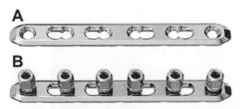

Fig. 2. LCP plates with sequential combi-holes that afford either cortical or locking screw fixation through the same hole. (Synthes, Paoli, PA, USA) (*Courtesy of* Jesse B. Jupiter, MD.)

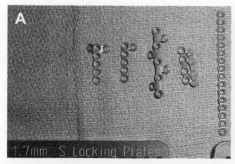
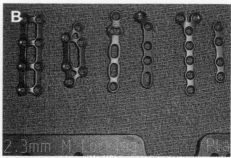
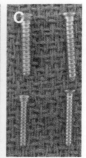

Fig. 3. Stryker VariAx hand locking module (Stryker-Leibinger, Kalamazoo, MI, USA) with (*A*) 1.7 mm and (*B*) 2.3 mm anatomically precontoured locking plates. (*C*) Locking (*left*) and nonlocking (*right*) screws are available for each screw hole: 2.3 mm (*top*), 1.7 mm (*bottom*). The grade 5 titanium alloy in the screw head obtains purchase within the screw hole made of softer grade 2 titanium to create the locking mechanism.

locking screws with compression washers can be placed through the compression hole to create axial compression (0.75 mm of compression per hole).

FIXATION BY ANATOMIC REGION
Distal Ulna

Unstable metaphyseal fractures of the distal ulna may be seen in up to 6% of patients with unstable fractures of the distal radius.[45] Optimal management of distal ulna articular head and/or metaphyseal neck fractures sustained in conjunction with an unstable distal radius fracture requiring operative fixation is not well established, and series reporting outcomes following operative treatment of these injuries remain limited.[45–50] Failure to achieve congruent anatomic reduction through stable fixation at the sigmoid notch and distal radioulnar joint (DRUJ) compromises the ability to reestablish ulnar variance and DRUJ stability, and thus increases the risk of distal ulna nonunion,[51–53] DRUJ dysfunction, ulnar-sided wrist pain, and posttraumatic arthrosis.[54]

Fixation of comminuted distal ulna head/neck fractures remains technically challenging (**Fig. 6**). Only 2 series have been published reporting results with angular-stable implants (2.0-mm, 2.4-mm, or 2.7-mm minicondylar blade plates,[49] or minifragment Y-, T-, or L-shaped locked plates)[46] for obtaining fixation within small, osteopenic, metaphyseal fragments and the short nonarticular arc of the ulnar head. Ring and colleagues.[49] reported good-to-excellent results in most of their cohort at a mean of 26 months following operative fixation of unstable distal ulna fractures with a minicondylar blade plate construct. Dennison[46] reported good-to-excellent radiographic alignment and clinical results in 5 patients following locked plating of an unstable distal ulna fracture at the time of operative fixation of a concomitant distal radius fracture.

In the distal ulna, exposure is achieved through the extensor carpi ulnaris–flexor carpi ulnaris interval, and the dorsal sensory branch of the ulnar nerve is identified and protected. When applying an angular-stable implant to the distal ulna, it is

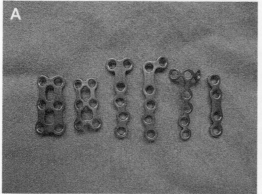
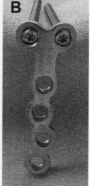

Fig. 4. The Medartis (Basel, Switzerland) Aptus titanium system: (*A*) screw holes are offset to reduce screw collision during polyaxial locking within a 15° cone and to avoid fracture propagation with drilling. (*B*) Locking is achieved through a TriLock radial 3-point wedge-locking mechanism.

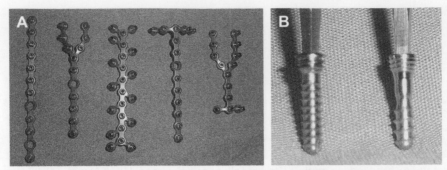

Fig. 5. (*A*) DePuy (Warsaw, IN, USA) titanium anatomic locked plating system (ALPS) with precontoured plating options. (*B*) Cobalt-chrome locking screws have polyaxial locking capabilities in this system.

helpful to identify the distal end of the ulna head under fluoroscopy to avoid plate or screw impingement on the triangular fibrocartilaginous complex. A Kirschner wire can be inserted from ulnar to radial deep to the triangular fibrocartilaginous complex to mark the distal extent that the plate may be applied. A 2.0-mm plate is appropriate in most patients, but a 2.4-mm or 2.7-mm plate may be selected in larger patients. The T-, Y-, or L-shaped terminal ends

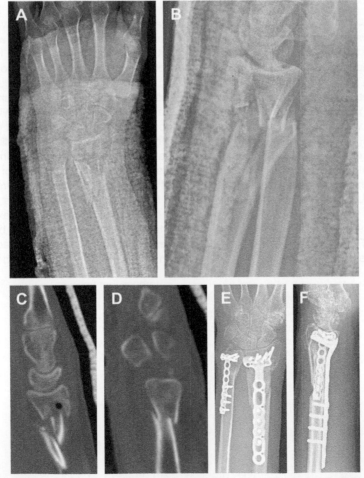

Fig. 6. (*A*) Posteroanterior and (*B*) lateral injury radiographs of a distal radius metadiaphyseal fracture with concomitant ulna neck and styloid fractures. (*C, D*) Corresponding images from the preoperative sagittal plane computed tomography reconstructions. (*E*) Postoperative posteroanterior and (*F*) lateral radiographs following plating of both fractures. (*Courtesy of* Chaitanya S. Mudgal, MD.)

of the locking plate are contoured with plate benders to anatomically fit the ulnar head segment. Contouring the plate to wrap around the ulnar head also helps to create orthogonal fixation, wherein the screws interlock in multiple planes to increase construct stability. Cannulated locking guides should be seated within the locking plate holes to prevent disruption of the locking mechanism as the plate is contoured. In the Synthes system (Paoli, PA, USA), the plate bending irons actually lock into the plate, thereby mimicking the locking guide and avoiding screw hole deformation.

The plate is secured to the distal ulna in an extraperiosteal fashion. Alternatively, if a minicondylar blade plate is selected, the track for the blade is drilled under fluoroscopic guidance. The blade length is determined and the blade is then cut to the measured length. Following insertion of the blade, the screw adjacent to the blade is inserted to compress the plate to the bone. The proximal screw holes are then filled.

If the metaphyseal neck is highly comminuted, nonlocking screws are placed in neutral positions to avoid compression through the zone of comminution. Unicortical locking screws are advantageous in the ulna head segment given its short nonarticular arc. Unicortical screws help to avoid articular penetration and subsequent impingement on the sigmoid notch during forearm rotation. In addition, supplemental locked screws along the construct help prevent loosening in osteoporotic bone.

Despite the availability of angular-stable locked plating fixation constructs[46,49] for distal ulnar articular/metaphyseal fractures, nonanatomic reduction,[45,46] loss of fixation in multifragmentary fractures, and symptomatic hardware necessitating additional surgery[49] remain significant problems with these fracture patterns.

Metacarpal and Phalangeal Shaft Fractures

Diaphyseal fractures of the metacarpals and phalanges may be multifragmentary, associated with significant cortical comminution, and show intercalary bone loss (**Fig. 7**). These fractures may occur in combined volar and/or dorsal skeletal and soft-tissue injuries. In addition, multiple ipsilateral consecutive metacarpal[55] or phalangeal fractures may be seen following significant trauma and necessitate rigid plate fixation. Goals of operative fixation include stable restoration of length, alignment, and axial rotation so that mobilization of injured structures can be initiated in the early postoperative period to maximize outcomes in patients with these complex combined injuries.

In these settings, locking plates appropriately sized for the injured region may be used to obtain stable fixation. Angular-stable plates applied with a bridging technique across the comminuted area avoid periosteal stripping and preserve vascularity. If corticocancellous bone graft is indicated, additional screw fixation can be placed to secure the graft. In the metacarpals, a paratendinous or extensor splitting exposure is used. In the border metacarpals, plate application may be dorsal or lateral. A dorsal or midaxial approach may be used in phalanges for lateral plate application. Biomechanical analyses[56,57] in cadaveric specimens have suggested that midlateral plate positioning may have superior biomechanical properties.

Periarticular Fractures

Phalangeal condylar fractures are typically unstable fracture patterns. The collateral ligament origin rotates the condylar fragment creating articular incongruity and angular deformity. Unicondylar fractures that are comminuted in the phalangeal neck region as well as bicondylar fractures may not be amendable to lag screw or Kirschner wire fixation techniques. For open reduction internal fixation, the interval between the central slip and lateral band or reflection of the central slip[58] is used. For these injuries a 1.5-mm minicondylar locking plate or blade plate[39,40] provides angular-stable fixation and subchondral support and allows for early postoperative rehabilitation. Combi-holes additionally allow for lag screw fixation of condylar fragments through the plate. These plates may be applied dorsally or laterally for juxtaarticular fractures.[39,40,59] The collateral ligament should be avoided when possible with lateral plate application to preserve the vascular supply to the condylar fragment and avoid mechanical impingement. Freeland and colleagues[60] have suggested that unilateral excision of the lateral band and oblique retinacular fibers of the metacarpophalangeal joint extensor expansion may decrease the risk of postoperative adhesions, tissue irritation, and intrinsic tightness when minicondylar plates are inserted on the lateral aspect of the proximal phalanx.

Injuries occurring at the base of the phalanx may be epibasilar/extraarticular or intraarticular. Exposure is performed through a paratendinous or tendon-splitting approach. When there is articular impaction, the articular surface is elevated by working through an adjacent fracture line. Provisional articular reduction is secured with Kirschner wires. T- or Y-shaped locking plates may be applied dorsally. The angular-stable screws

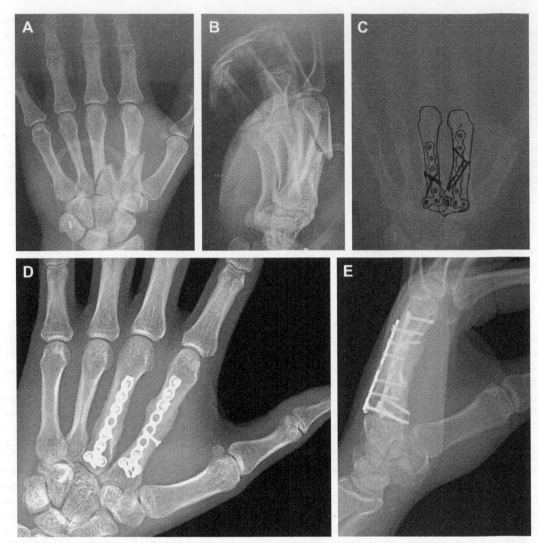

Fig. 7. (*A*) Posteroanterior and (*B*) lateral injury radiographs of high-energy ipsilateral index and long-finger metacarpal fractures. The index metacarpal fracture shows multifragmentary metadiaphyseal comminution and the long-finger metacarpal is epibasilar. (*C*) Preoperative template showing a 2.0-mm plate applied in a bridging mode across the area of comminution in the index metacarpal. In the long-finger metacarpal, the 2.0-mm plate is used as a neutralization plate following application of a 2.0-mm cortical lag screw. (*D*) Postoperative posteroanterior and (*E*) lateral radiographs at latest follow-up show anatomic alignment and fracture union. (*Courtesy of* Chaitanya S. Mudgal, MD.)

through the periarticular position of the plate serve to optimize metaphyseal fixation (**Fig. 8**) and buttress the elevated articular surface when there has been joint impaction. As with nonlocked plates, malrotation and malalignment may occur if only a single screw is placed in the periarticular portion of the plate and a shaft screw is placed with the plate eccentrically placed on the diaphysis.

In select cases, intraarticular fractures at the base of the thumb (ie, epibasilar, Bennett, and Rolando fractures) and the fifth metacarpal may be treated with open reduction and internal fixation. Dorsally applied angular-stable implants resist flexion deformity at the fracture site created by comminution on the volar cortex. In addition, improved metaphyseal fixation is achieved. For 3-part articular fractures (ie, Rolando fractures), the site of plate application is selected after careful analysis of the fracture pattern in the coronal and sagittal planes. Articular restoration is attempted with lag screw fixation. Alternatively, nonlocked

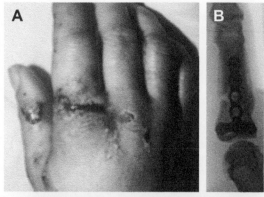

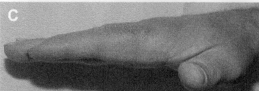

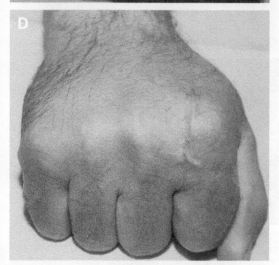

Fig. 8. (*A*) Combined injury to index finger which included an open fracture of the proximal phalanx at the metadiaphyseal junction. (*B*) Dorsal plating of the proximal phalanx fracture allowed for early range of motion following this combined injury and osseous union. (*C, D*) Functional range of motion was achieved at latest follow-up. (*Courtesy of* Chaitanya S. Mudgal, MD.)

screws may be placed eccentrically in the condylar segment of the plate to create compression of the articular fracture line. These can then be replaced with locked screws.

Delayed Reconstruction: Nonunion, Osteotomy, and Arthrodesis in the Hand

Nonunions and malunions of the metacarpals and phalanges continue to represent unique challenges for the hand surgeon. Angular and rotational deformity with functional deficits are indications for surgical correction. Previous scars and tendon adhesions may make exposure challenging, and the presence of soft-tissue contractures may increase the stress on the fixation. In the setting of these complex non- and malunions, angular-stable fixation may allow early functional rehabilitation following concomitant tenolysis, arthrolysis, and capsulectomy.

Nonunions of the tubular bones of the hand are uncommon. There are limited reports of the results of treatment of metacarpal and phalangeal non- and malunions.[61,62] Jupiter and colleagues,[61] in a series of 25 nonunions/delayed unions, found plate and screw fixation achieved a more functional digit compared with several other techniques. Implant selection depends on the location and direction of the non-/malunion within the longitudinal axis of the involved bone. Diaphyseal corrections are amenable to straight plates or extended H-plates. In transverse nonunions, cortical screws can be used to achieve compression across the nonunion site before placing locking screws (**Fig. 9**). Minicondylar plates are used for metaphyseal, juxtarticular, or combined metadiaphyseal reconstructions. As a general rule, in the setting of these reconstructions, implants one size larger than would be required for an acute fracture at the same level should be considered (ie, 2.4-mm plates in the metacarpal and 2.0-mm plates in the proximal phalanx). The need for intercalary structural corticocancellous grafting is determined preoperatively. Additional locking screws can be used to stabilize the graft at the nonunion or osteotomy site.

When corrective osteotomy is performed at the site of the original fracture, a complex multiplanar deformity can be completely addressed while simultaneously performing tenolysis and arthrolysis. Buchler and colleagues[63] reported good-to-excellent results in 96% of patients following corrective osteotomy for isolated posttraumatic phalangeal malunions; however, this rate dropped to 64% when soft-tissue structures were also involved. In this setting, rigid fixation is required to allow for early postoperative rehabilitation to optimize outcome.

Arthrodesis represents a salvage option for the stiff painful joint adjacent to a periarticular nonunion. Various fixation techniques have been described for arthrodesis in the hand. Use of angular-stable fixation allows the surgeon to use a single construct to address the nonunion site (ie, debridement, bone grafting, and fixation) while concomitantly providing for stability at the involved joint to achieve solid fusion.

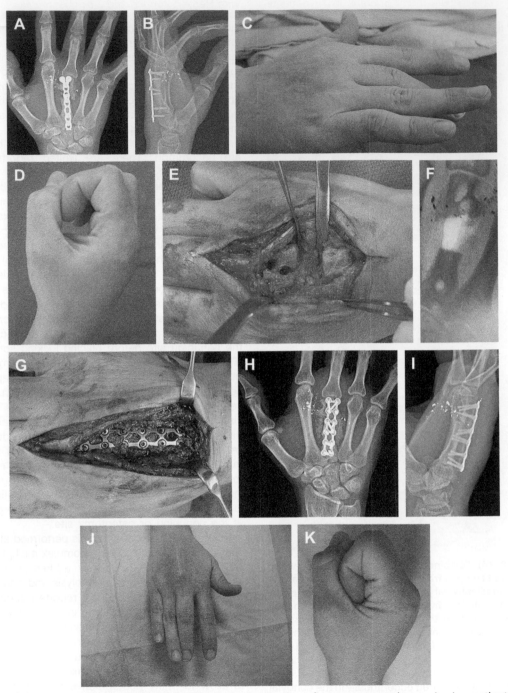

Fig. 9. (*A*) Posteroanterior and (*B*) lateral radiographs showing long-finger metacarpal nonunion in a patient who suffered a low velocity gun shot wound, followed by multiple unsuccessful attempts at achieving union. (*C, D*) Preoperative clinical examination demonstrated digital stiffness and extrinsic tightness. (*E*) Intraoperative image following removal of hardware and debridement of the nonunion site. (*F*) Corresponding intraoperative fluoroscopic image of the segmental bone gap following debridement of the nonunion site. (*G*) Intraoperative image following iliac crest autograft and hybrid fixation using a combination of locked and nonlocked screws. Maximal fixation was obtained by using an extended H-plate. (*H*) Posteroanterior and (*I*) lateral radiographs following nonunion repair. (*J, K*) An excellent clinical outcome was achieved. (*Courtesy of* Chaitanya S. Mudgal, MD.)

COMPLICATIONS

The complications reported following plating of metacarpal and phalangeal fractures[3,40] are also seen following the use of locked plates in the hand. However, several complications are unique to locking technology. The locked screws can disengage from the plate secondary to failure of the screw to seat into the plate properly because of cross-threading (where the screw threads and the plate threads are not collinear) or when insufficient screw torque is used to engage the screw head into the plate in systems relying on alternate methods of locking. The screws can break or disengage from the plate under excessive cyclical loading. Despite an excellent feel intraoperatively, locked plates may cease providing fragment fixation as a result of exceedingly poor bone quality, excessive comminution, or suboptimal plate length to working length ratio.

Nonunion and malunion can still occur with the use of locked plates if anatomic contouring is imprecisely performed. The locking sleeves provided in select systems should be secured within the locking screw holes when plate contouring is required to prevent disruption of the locking mechanism. In addition, locked screws should only be placed after a direct anatomic reduction is achieved. Placement of locked screws before reduction confers malreduction that is not correctable.

When a hybrid construct is used with locked screws placed to augment compression plating, it is essential to achieve maximal compression across the fracture site with standard cortical non-locking screws before the insertion of locked screws. When locked screws are placed on both sides of the fracture before fracture compression, fracture gap will result. This scenario increases fracture site strain and implant stresses, and may lead to nonunion and/or hardware failure.

SUMMARY

Locked fixed-angle plating in the hand and wrist will continue to evolve. This technology is most appropriate in acute fractures or reconstructions with long plate working lengths, short periarticular segments, and the absence of bony support on the contralateral cortex from the side of plate application. Clinical experience with locking technology in hand trauma remains relatively limited compared with its application in larger extremity long bones. A thorough understanding of the biomechanics and fracture personality are required to apply fixed-angle plates correctly, optimize outcomes, and avoid iatrogenic nonunion and malunion.

REFERENCES

1. Dabezies EJ, Schutte JP. Fixation of metacarpal and phalangeal fractures with miniature plates and screws. J Hand Surg Am 1986;11(2):283–8.
2. Hastings H. Unstable metacarpal and phalangeal fracture treatment with screws and plates. Clin Orthop Relat Res 1987;214:37–52.
3. Page SM, Stern PJ. Complications and range of motion following plate fixation of metacarpal and phalangeal fractures. J Hand Surg 1998;23:827–32.
4. Stern PJ. Management of fractures of the hand over the last 25 years. J Hand Surg 2000;25:817–23.
5. Handschin AE, Cardell M, Contaldo C, et al. Functional results of angular-stable plate fixation in displaced proximal humeral fractures. Injury 2008;39:306–13.
6. Egol KA, Ong CC, Walsh M, et al. Early complications in proximal humerus fractures (OTA Types 11) treated with locked plates. J Orthop Trauma 2008;22(3):159–64.
7. Gardner MJ, Weil Y, Barker JU, et al. The importance of medial support in locked plating of proximal humerus fractures. J Orthop Trauma 2007;21(3):185–91.
8. Koukakis A, Apostolou CD, Taneja T, et al. Fixation of proximal humerus fractures using the PHILOS plate: early experience. Clin Orthop Relat Res 2006;442:115–20.
9. Tejwani NC, Murthy A, Park J, et al. Fixation of extra-articular distal humerus fractures using one locking plate versus two reconstruction plates: a laboratory study. J Trauma 2009;66(3):795–9.
10. Jupiter JB, Marent-Huber M, LCP Study Group. Operative management of distal radial fractures with 2.4-millimeter locking plates. A multicenter prospective case series. J Bone Joint Surg Am 2009;91(1):55–65.
11. Orbay JL, Fernandez DL. Volar fixation for dorsally displaced fractures of the distal radius: a preliminary report. J Hand Surg Am 2002;27:205–15.
12. Mudgal CS, Jupiter JB. Plate fixation of osteoporotic fractures of the distal radius. J Orthop Trauma 2008;22(Suppl 8):S106–15.
13. Koshimune M, Kamano M, Takamatsu K, et al. A randomized comparison of locking and non-locking palmar plating for unstable Colles' fractures in the elderly. J Hand Surg Br 2005;30:499–503.
14. Chung KC, Watt AJ, Kotsis SV, et al. Treatment of unstable distal radial fractures with the volar locking plating system. J Bone Joint Surg Am 2006;88:2687–94.
15. Fankhauser F, Gruber G, Schippinger G, et al. Minimal-invasive treatment of distal femoral fractures with the LISS (Less Invasive Stabilization System): a prospective study of 30 fractures with

a follow up of 20 months. Acta Orthop Scand 2004; 75:56–60.

16. Kregor PJ, Stannard JA, Zlowodzki M, et al. Treatment of distal femur fractures using the less invasive stabilization system: surgical experience and early clinical results in 103 fractures. J Orthop Trauma 2004;18:509–20.

17. Buttaro MA, Farfalli G, Paredes-Nunez M, et al. Locking compression plate fixation of Vancouver type-B1 periprosthetic femoral fractures. J Bone Joint Surg Am 2007;89:1964–9.

18. Erhardt JB, Grob K, Roderer G, et al. Treatment of periprosthetic femur fractures with the non-contact bridging plate: a new angular stable implant. Arch Orthop Trauma Surg 2008;128:409–16.

19. Gosling T, Schandelmaier P, Muller M, et al. Single lateral locked screw plating of bicondylar tibial plateau fractures. Clin Orthop Relat Res 2005;439: 207–14.

20. Ricci WM, Rudzki JR, Borrelli J Jr. Treatment of complex proximal tibia fractures with the less invasive skeletal stabilization system. J Orthop Trauma 2004;18:521–7.

21. Bahari S, Lenehan B, Khan H, et al. Minimally invasive percutaneous plate fixation of distal tibia fractures. Acta Orthop Belg 2007;73:635–40.

22. Lozano-Calderón S, Moore M, Liebman M, et al. Distal radius osteotomy in the elderly patient using angular stable implants and Norian bone cement. J Hand Surg Am 2007;32(7):976–83.

23. Malone KJ, Magnell TD, Freeman DC, et al. Surgical correction of dorsally angulated distal radius malunions with fixed angle volar plating: a case series. J Hand Surg Am 2006;3:366–72.

24. Cordey J, Borgeaud M, Perren SM. Force transfer between the plate and the bone: relative importance of the bending stiffness of the screws friction between plate and bone. Injury 2000;31(Suppl 3):C21–8.

25. Cordey J, Mikuschka-Galgoczy E, Blumlein H, et al. Importance of the friction between plate and bone in the anchoring of plates for osteosynthesis: determination of the coefficient of metal-bone friction in animal in vivo. Helv Chir Acta 1979;46:183–7.

26. Simon JA, Dennis MG, Kummer FJ, et al. Schuhli augmentation of plate and screw fixation for humeral shaft fractures: a laboratory study. J Orthop Trauma 1999;13:196–9.

27. Ramotowski W, Granowski R. Zespol. An original method of stable osteosynthesis. Clin Orthop Relat Res 1991;272:67–75.

28. Borgeaud M, Cordey J, Leyvraz PE, et al. Mechanical analysis of the bone to plate interface of the LC-DCP and of the PC-FIX on human femora. Injury 2000;31(Suppl 3):C29–36.

29. Eijer H, Hauke C, Arens S, et al. PC-Fix and local infection resistance—influence of implant design on postoperative infection development, clinical

and experimental results. Injury 2001;32(Suppl 2): B38–43.

30. Cole PA, Zlowodzki M, Kregor PJ. Less Invasive Stabilization System (LISS) for fractures of the proximal tibia: indications, surgical technique and preliminary results of the UMC Clinical Trial. Injury 2003;34(Suppl 1):A16–29.

31. Frigg R, Appenzeller A, Christensen R, et al. The development of the distal femur Less Invasive Stabilization System (LISS). Injury 2001;32(Suppl 3): SC24–31.

32. Goesling T, Frenk A, Appenzeller A, et al. Liss Plt: design, mechanical and biomechanical characteristics. Injury 2003;34(Suppl 1):A11–5.

33. Haidukewych GJ. Innovations in locking plate technology. J Am Acad Orthop Surg 2004;12:205–12.

34. Gardner MJ, Lorich DG, Werner CM, et al. Second-generation concepts for locked plating of proximal humerus fractures. Am J Orthop 2007;36(9):460–5.

35. Egol KA, Kubiak EN, Fulkerson E, et al. Biomechanics of locked plates and screws. J Orthop Trauma 2004;18:488–93.

36. Gardner MJ, Helfet DL, Lorich DG. Has locked plating completely replaced conventional plating? Am J Orthop 2004;33:439–46.

37. Perren SM. Evolution of the internal fixation of long bone fractures. The scientific basis of biological internal fixation: choosing a new balance between stability and biology. J Bone Joint Surg Br 2002;84: 1093–110.

38. Shyamalan G, Theokli C, Pearse Y, et al. Volar locking plates versus Kirschner wires for distal radial fractures – a cost analysis study. Injury 2009;40: 1279–81.

39. Büchler U, Fischer T. Use of a minicondylar plate for metacarpal and phalangeal periarticular injuries. Clin Orthop Relat Res 1987;214:53–8.

40. Ouellette EA, Freeland AE. Use of the minicondylar plate in metacarpal and phalangeal fractures. Clin Orthop Relat Res 1996;327:38–46.

41. Damron TA, Jebson PJ, Rao VK, et al. Biomechanical analysis of dorsal plate fixation in proximal phalangeal fractures. Ann Plast Surg 1994;32(3): 270–5.

42. Nunley JA, Kloen P. Biomechanical and functional testing of plate fixation devices for proximal phalangeal fractures. J Hand Surg Am 1991;16(6):991–8.

43. Prevel CD, Eppley BL, Jackson JR, et al. Mini and micro plating of phalangeal and metacarpal fractures: a biomechanical study. J Hand Surg Am 1995;20(1):44–9.

44. Leibovic SJ. Internal fixation sets for use in the hand. A comparison of available instrumentation. Hand Clin 1997;13(4):531–40.

45. Biyani A, Simison AJ, Klenerman L. Fractures of the distal radius and ulna. J Hand Surg Br 1995;20(3): 357–64.

Intramedullary Nail Fixation for Metacarpal Fractures

Philip E. Blazar, MD*, Dante Leven

KEYWORDS

- Metacarpal fractures • Treatment • Surgical techniques
- Intramedullary nail fixation

Fractures of the metacarpals are among the most common types of fractures involving the upper extremity. Multiple studies have reported that these fractures account for approximately 10% of all fractures.[1–5] Their ubiquitous nature warrants a complete understanding of the anatomy, fracture patterns, proper evaluation, and treatment options by the orthopedist. These fractures usually can be managed nonsurgically; although patient age, occupation, medical health, and activity level must be considered when reviewing surgical indications. These fractures occur more commonly in men, and the peak incidence occurs in the age group of 10 to 40 years, when involvement in athletics and occupation peaks. In addition, technological advancements have revolutionized the treatment of metacarpal fractures, for which complicated fracture patterns once posed a significant challenge to the surgeon and the patient. Various surgical options exist for the treatment of metacarpal fractures when surgery is indicated, including open or closed reduction with Kirschner wire (K-wire) fixation; open reduction internal fixation with plates and/or screws; and more recently, intramedullary nail (IMN) fixation.

APPLIED ANATOMY

The metacarpals extend from the carpus to the proximal phalanges. The ulnar metacarpals form the longitudinal and transverse arches of the hand with their concave palmar alignment and the increasing mobility in the palmar direction of the more ulnar metacarpals. Ligamentous support at the carpometacarpal (CMC) joint is restrictive, allowing minimal clinical motion at the index and long CMC joints and up to 30° or 40° of flexion or extension motion in the small finger. The ligaments supporting the condyloid-shaped metacarpophalangeal (MCP) joints allow flexion, extension, abduction, adduction, and circumduction. The collateral ligaments, taut in flexion as a result of the cam shape of the metacarpal head, support the MCP joints in the sagittal plane. The volar plates resist hyperextension at this joint, and adjacent plates are connected by the transverse intercarpal ligaments. The small finger and ring finger CMC joints articulate with the hamate, the middle finger with the capitate, the index finger with the trapezoid, and the thumb with the trapezium.

SURGICAL CONSIDERATIONS

Anatomic considerations are important for defining the fracture pattern as well as determining the optimal treatment approach. The fracture location is important and typically described as metacarpal head, neck, shaft, or base. The normal neck-to-shaft angle of 15° is important to consider when reviewing radiographs. Fractures of the metacarpal neck are the most common, whereas fractures of the metacarpal head are relatively uncommon and usually intra-articular. Metacarpal shaft fractures are described as transverse, oblique, or comminuted. When angulation is present, the ring and small fingers can generally tolerate more angulation than the long and index fingers because of the increased CMC mobility of these

Department of Orthopaedics Surgery, Brigham and Women's Hospital, 75 Francis Street, Boston, MA 02115, USA
* Corresponding author.
E-mail address: pblazar@partners.org

Hand Clin 26 (2010) 321–325
doi:10.1016/j.hcl.2010.05.005

rays. Some investigators suggest that angulation greater than 40° at the small finger, 30° at the ring finger, and 15° at the long and index finger is unacceptable.[1,2]

Most metacarpal fractures occur with an axial load directed proximally through the MCP joint and result in a transverse fracture, with the fracture apex forming dorsally. This dorsal angulation occurs because of the interossei muscle origins along the metacarpals. With a torsional force, the fracture becomes oblique or spiral and the fracture may comminute with high-energy trauma. Rotational deformity can occur, depending on the direction and quantity of force involved.[5]

Consideration of surrounding soft tissue structures is also critical and may influence surgical management. Vascular, tendon, nerve, or skin damage must be assessed and may often indicate surgical exploration. Only a thin soft tissue envelope exists along the dorsal surface of the hand. Significant infection can occur through seemingly trivial soft tissue wounds, particularly in cases of contamination by oral flora from fight bites. Similarly, the extensor tendons are intimately opposed to the dorsal surface of the metacarpals and are apt to injury.

Although metacarpal fractures can often be managed nonoperatively, indications for surgery include irreducible fractures; malrotation; displaced intra-articular fractures; open fractures; segmental bone loss; associated soft tissue injuries; and angulation of greater than 15° in the index and long fingers, greater than 30° in the ring finger, and greater than 40° in the small finger.

Examination often supersedes radiographic measurements in detecting single metacarpal fractures. For instance, marked shortening and rotational deformity are widely accepted surgical indications, whereas sagittal angular deformity needs to be severe enough that the surgeon considers it likely to result in unacceptable alignment and function. Fractures involving multiple metacarpals are typically indicated for surgery even with minimal displacement or angulation at presentation, because the anatomic stability gained from the adjacent transverse intercarpal ligaments is usually corrupted.

INTRAMEDULLARY NAIL FIXATION

Intramedullary fixation of metacarpal shaft and the neck fractures with K-wires has been used with success.[3] However, intramedullary K-wire fixation does not always provide rigid fixation and may allow some degree of angulation to develop. This technique is also less useful in cases of rotational deformity or spiral or comminuted fractures.

K-wire fixation is typically indicated in transverse or oblique fractures. This technique can also be used in cases involving more than one metacarpal fracture, although relative to more stable methods of fixation, instituting early motion may be difficult. Faraj and Davis[3] suggest burying the intramedullary K-wire in the metacarpal rather than cutting it flush or leaving a small portion protruding, to prevent retraction and subsequent soft tissue impingement. These investigators also recommend placing the cortical window at least 1 cm distal to the CMC joint to prevent encroachment into the articular space.

Intramedullary nailing with prebent implants can be performed in a locked or nonlocked manner. Theoretically, 3-point fixation is achieved in any direction with this implant, although there are no biomechanical studies documenting the added stability. The implant comes in 2 sizes, with a diameter of 0.062 or 0.045 in. It has a blunt prebent tip and comes on a handheld inserter along with a bending device and a cap for locking.

Small Bone Fixation System

There is limited literature available addressing in detail the indications for the small bone fixation system (Depuy/Hand Innovations, Miami, FL, USA) type of fixation in comparison with the other alternatives. There is also little information on the additional stability afforded by the locking mechanism over nonlocking fixation. The potential advantage over internal fixation with plates or interfragmentary screws is less soft tissue dissection and avoidance of late hardware removal, as well as potential decrease for extensor tendon irritation from metal. IMN fixation is recommended primarily for displaced metacarpal shaft fractures that are transverse or oblique (**Fig. 1**) and if there is an indication for surgery. Fractures with butterfly fragments and/or comminution are also amenable to this form of fixation; however, longitudinal fracture collapse can be seen. Open and multiple metacarpal fractures can be treated as well. In the authors' experience, fractures that are in the metadiaphyseal region either proximally or distally are less amenable to this form of fixation.

SURGICAL TECHNIQUE

Intraoperative fluoroscopy is required for IMN fixation. Regional anesthesia is preferred, but multiple options exist depending on the medical comorbidities and patient preferences. An arm tourniquet may be applied but is rarely required. For fractures in the middle or distal shaft, the entry is in the proximal metaphyseal region. For proximal third shaft fractures, a distal metaphyseal entry is used.

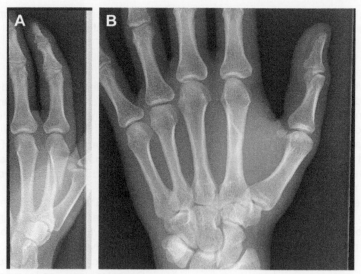

Fig. 1. Preoperative (*A*) oblique and (*B*) posteroanterior radiographs of the injury.

Implants come in 2 sizes; in the authors' experience, the largest size typically fits in most cases. A stab incision is made over the appropriate metaphyseal flare, and blunt dissection is carried down to the bone. The awl is introduced into the medullary canal by hand; the procedure is typically easy even in patients with thick cortical bone. A common error is to introduce the awl past the appropriate point. Fluoroscopy is used to confirm the appropriate placement of the awl into the medullary canal in 2 planes, and the nail is introduced through the cannulated awl into the medullary canal. The nail is advanced across the fracture site under fluoroscopic guidance. Use of a mallet to advance the nail can be helpful but typically, if the nail is in the correct position, it advances with little difficulty. The nail is advanced into the metaphyseal bone at the opposite end of the metacarpal and firmly seated. To avoid cutout, the nail should not be seated excessively distal across the distal metaphysis (**Fig. 2**). After confirming clinical and fluoroscopic alignment, the nail is bent at the entry point with the supplied benders and cut short. It has not been the authors' practice to lock these implants, but other investigators do so. The implant can be cut short and the end

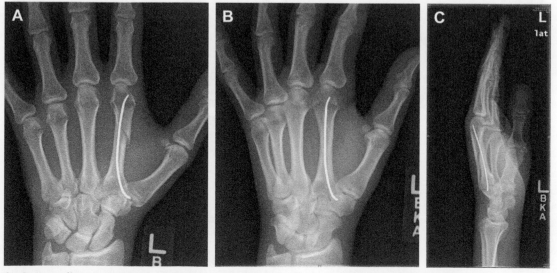

Fig. 2. Immediate postoperative (*A*) posteroanterior, (*B*) oblique, and (*C*) lateral radiographs.

buried, or it can be left percutaneous for later removal. When the implant is left percutaneously, removal requires more manipulation than with standard K-wires because of the 3-dimensional geometry, and therefore the authors' preference would be to remove these implants after sedation. Further technical details are available in a recent article by Orbay and Touhami.[6]

A range of motion exercises are initiated under the supervision of a hand therapist at the first postoperative visit and a forearm-based splint is typically worn for 4 weeks (**Fig. 3**). Union is typically seen clinically and radiographically at 4 to 6 weeks (**Fig. 4**) and, if needed, passive range of motion and strengthening exercises are begun. Implant removal can be done at union, similar to percutaneous fixation, or may be delayed if the implants are buried.

COMPLICATIONS

The complications of internal fixation with an intramedullary device are similar in type to those of other surgical treatments with internal fixation; specifically nonunion and malunion, superficial and deep infections, stiffness, hardware migration, stiffness, and tendon adhesions. Tendon rupture from prominent hardware has been reported. Implant migration through subchondral bone or "backing out" and implant fracture have been reported.[1,2] The senior author has seen delayed union and metacarpal shortening occur as well

as percutaneously placed implants developing pin tract infections.

DISCUSSION

Fracture patterns investigated in the literature include extra-articular oblique and transverse fractures, and generally involve either the metacarpal diaphysis or metaphysis. An anterograde approach is taken for fractures of the distal third of the metacarpal shaft, whereas fractures of the proximal third are approached in a retrograde manner.

It is important to realize that there is literature reviewing similar techniques using multiple hand-bent K-wires to provide fixation. This technique typically involves the insertion of several flexible implants, which are buried. A retrospective study by Gonzalez and colleagues[2] assessed the outcomes of 98 metacarpal fractures at 5 years postoperatively. All fractures were oblique or transverse and treated with flexible IMN using 0.8-mm prebent nails. Three complications occurred, including bending of the nail with repeated trauma in 2 cases and retraction of the rod in 1 case.

In a study by Ozer and colleagues,[1] IMN was compared with plate and screw fixation for extra-articular metacarpal fractures in 52 patients. The study was not randomized. IMN was performed without insertion of the available locking device. Operative time was much shorter in the IMN group; 15 minutes compared with 34 minutes for

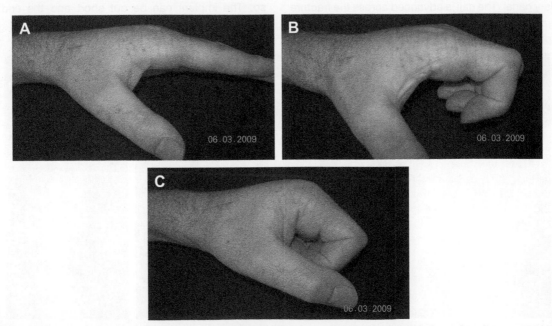

Fig. 3. Clinical images (*A, B, C*) of the active range of motion at union approximately 6 weeks postoperatively.

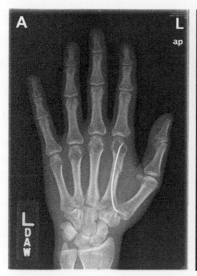 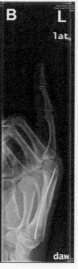 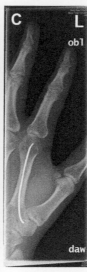

Fig. 4. Six weeks postoperative (*A*) posteroanterior, (*B*) lateral, and (*C*) oblique radiographs.

the plate and screw fixation technique. Hardware removal was not routinely considered. No statistical postoperative difference was found in total active motion, Disabilities of the Arm, Shoulder and Hand (DASH) scores, or radiographic parameters at follow-up. In particular, there was no difference in radiographic parameters except for 5 cases of implant migration in the IMN group, which were revised to plate and screw fixation. However, the investigators did note a higher incidence of tendon irritation, and cases requiring removal of hardware in 15 of 38 cases in the IMN group in contrast to 2 of 14 cases in the plate and screw fixation group.[1] The investigators concluded that the majority of the increases in complications were related to fractures in the distal third of the metacarpal, and did not recommend the use of the implant in that group.

SUMMARY

In the authors' experience, IMN fixation has proven to be reliable for select transverse and oblique metacarpal fractures (including multiple metacarpal fractures) for which surgery is indicated. The procedure is technically less challenging than open reduction and internal fixation with plates and screws, and early range of movement and return to occupational and recreational activities is possible. Like all procedures complications do exist, but careful surgical technique can minimize these risks. Implant removal is commonly required.

REFERENCES

1. Ozer K, Gillani S, Williams A. Comparison of intramedullary nailing versus plate-screw fixation of extra-articular metacarpal fractures. J Hand Surg Am 2008;33(10):1724–31.
2. Gonzalez MH, Igram CM, Hall RF Jr. Flexible intramedullary nailing for metacarpal fractures. J Hand Surg Am 1995;20:382–7.
3. Faraj A, Davis T. Percutaneous intramedullary fixation of metacarpal shaft fractures. J Hand Surg Br 1999; 24(1):76–9.
4. Kaiser MM, Tafazzoli K, Theilen TM, et al. Intramedullary nailing for metacarpal 2-5 fractures. J Pediatr Orthop B 2009 Jul 17. [Epub ahead of print].
5. Manueddu CA, Della Santa D. Fasciculated intramedullary pinning of metacarpal fractures. J Hand Surg Br 1996;21. p. 230–6.
6. Orbay JL, Touhami A. The treatment of unstable metacarpal and phalangeal shaft fractures with flexible non-locking and locking intramedullary nails. Hand Clin 2006;22:279–86.

the plate and screw fixation technique. Hardware removal was not routinely considered. No statistical postoperative difference was found in total active motion, Disabilities of the Arm, Shoulder and Hand (DASH) scores, or radiographic parameters at follow-up. In particular, there was no difference in radiographic parameters except for 5 cases of implant migration in the IMN group, which were revised to plate and screw fixation. However, the investigators did note a higher incidence of tendon irritation and cases requiring removal of hardware in 15 of 59 cases in the IMN group in contrast to 2 of 14 cases in the plate and screw fixation group. The investigators concluded that the majority of the increases in complications were related to fractures in the distal third of the metacarpal and did not recommend the use of the implant in that group.

SUMMARY

In the authors' experience, IMN fixation has proven to be reliable to select transverse and oblique metacarpal fractures, (including irreducible metacarpal fractures) for which surgery is indicated. The procedure is technically less challenging than open reduction and internal fixation with plates and screws, and early range of movement and return to occupational and recreational activities is possible. Like all procedures, complications do exist, but careful surgical technique can minimize these risks. Implant removal is commonly required.

REFERENCES

Implant Arthroplasty of the Carpometacarpal Joint of the Thumb

David J. Bozentka, MD[a,b,*]

KEYWORDS

- Thumb total joint arthroplasty • Trapeziometacarpal implant
- Arthritis • Carpometacarpal joint

Trapeziometacarpal arthritis is the second most common joint affected by degenerative arthritis.[1] Patients with the disorder develop pain, stiffness, and swelling at the base of the thumb, aggravated by activities of grasp, pinch, and fine manipulation. Initial treatment is nonoperative and includes splints, medications, corticosteroid injections, and activity modification. If nonoperative treatment modalities fail, multiple surgical options are available.

Surgical treatment of the arthritic thumb carpometacarpal joint is based on clinical staging of the disease, patient functional demand, and surgeon preference. Before the development of significant radiographic changes, such as Eaton stage I arthritis,[2] patients are treated with ligament reconstruction or metacarpal osteotomy. More advanced stages, Eaton stages II to IV, may be treated with resection arthroplasty with numerous variations.

The trapezium resection may be partial or complete and can be performed open or arthroscopically. Partial excision of the trapezium maintains thumb length, preserving pinch strength. This technique involves an interposition of autologous material, such as a harvested tendon, or nonautologous material. A ligament reconstruction using flexor carpi radialis or abductor pollicis longus for stabilization also can be considered. Complete trapeziectomy with or without ligament reconstruction and interposition provides pain relief,

although long-term studies have shown progressive shortening of the thumb with resultant weakness of lateral pinch strength.[3,4]

Trapeziometacarpal arthrodesis was first described by Muller[5] in 1949, and is considered for young patients with high functional demand. Limitations of thumb carpometacarpal arthrodesis include prolonged healing time, restricted motion, and the development of arthritis in adjacent joints, specifically the scaphoid trapezoid joint.[6,7]

In an effort to maintain motion, prevent thumb shortening, and improve pinch strength, while limiting postoperative recovery time, various thumb carpometacarpal implant arthroplasties have been developed. The goal when performing a thumb carpometacarpal arthroplasty is to obtain a pain-free, stable, mobile joint. The ideal thumb basal joint implant would restore the structure and function of the joint. Development of the ideal prosthesis similar to the anatomy of this complex joint while attaining the proposed goals is a difficult task. Trapeziometacarpal implants have been plagued with loosening, breakage, instability, and stiffness.[8]

Surgeons encounter multiple challenges in replacing the thumb carpometacarpal joint. The pinch forces at the pulp of the thumb are magnified 10 to 13 times at the thumb carpometacarpal level, leading to significant stress on the implant and increasing the risk of loosening.[9] The thumb carpometacarpal joint has no single center of rotation.

The author has nothing to disclose and no conflict relevant to the subject matter in the article.
[a] Department of Orthopedic Surgery, University of Pennsylvania School of Medicine, Second Floor Silverstein Pavilion, 3400 Spruce Street, Philadelphia, PA 19104, USA
[b] Department of Orthopedic Surgery, Penn Presbyterian Medical Center, 1 Cupp Pavilion, 39th and Market Street, Philadelphia, PA 19104, USA
* Department of Orthopedic Surgery, Penn Presbyterian Medical Center, 1 Cupp Pavilion, 39th and Market Street, Philadelphia, PA 19104.
E-mail address: David.bozentka@uphs.upenn.edu

Hand Clin 26 (2010) 327–337
doi:10.1016/j.hcl.2010.05.007

Thumb circumduction involves a combined multi-axial motion.[10] Instantaneous motion occurs between the centers of rotation for flexion and extension, and abduction and adduction. In addition, the arthritic thumb carpometacarpal joint is typically associated with a deformity, with dorsoradial displacement of the metacarpal on the trapezium. The poor soft tissues with capsular attenuation lead to the instability, and this preoperative subluxation must be addressed. The small bones, shallow joint contour with erosive changes, and angulation add to the technical difficulties.[11]

Multiple designs and materials have been used for implant arthroplasty of the thumb carpometacarpal joint but with varying success.[8] Initial thumb carpometacarpal joint implants made of silicone were popularized by Swanson and Niebauer and colleagues[12,13] in the 1960s. Later in the 1970s, ball-and-socket total joint prostheses with a metal metacarpal and polyethylene trapezium were developed similar to the total hip arthroplasty concept.[14] The most common complication of these prostheses, whether cemented or uncemented, is loosening.

Performing a trapeziometacarpal arthroplasty in the presence of scaphotrapezium–trapezoid (STT) joint arthritis is controversial. Advanced stages of arthritic changes in this location are a contraindication, although the procedure may be performed for patients with mild stages of STT arthritis. The joint is palpated preoperatively. Significant tenderness of the STT joint or severe radiographic changes of arthritis in this location are a contraindication for the procedure, in which case a resection arthroplasty should be considered.[15] Other contraindications include prior infection of the thumb carpometacarpal joint, a Charcot joint, or paralytic contracture of the hand.[16]

TOTAL JOINT ARTHROPLASTY

de la Caffiniere[17] presented the preliminary results of a cemented thumb carpometacarpal total joint arthroplasty. The stem design was later changed in 1991, making it more bulky proximally. The Caffiniere prosthesis is the most extensively used and studied total joint arthroplasty for the trapeziometacarpal joint. It is a semiconstrained articulated ball-and-socket joint. Both components are cemented, including a cobalt chromium metacarpal component and a polyethylene cup for the trapezium. The size of the trapezium must be adequate to accommodate the single-sized cup and a modest amount of methylmethacrylate. Intraoperatively, 2 to 4 mm of the base of the metacarpal is excised parallel to the metacarpophalangeal joint. Care must be taken to ensure minimal loss of bone stock and thumb length. The trapezium is reamed with a small burr, preserving a modest amount of cortical overhang to support the component and cement. After cement placement, the articulated components are inserted initially into the metacarpal. The cup is then seated in the radial-most part of the trapezium, maintaining it perpendicular to the rim of the trapezium. The thumb is immobilized for approximately 3 weeks to allow capsular healing, followed by graduated use.[18]

Boeckstyns and colleagues[19] reported their series of 31 implants in 28 patients with an average follow-up of 48 months and range 13 to 77 months. Four of the hands needed reoperation, including six cups and one metacarpal component. They found that removal of loose implants typically occurred early after implantation, and noted a 3-year survival rate of 90% and 5-year survival rate of 80%. At final follow-up 27 of the 29 patients available for assessment had no or slight pain, and the remaining 2 had moderate pain.

Hamlin[18] noted an approximately 7% failure rate, with failures typically involving breakdown of the bone–cement interface at the trapezium.

van Cappelle and colleagues[20] reported acceptable results in their series of 77 implants using the first-generation prosthesis. The average age was 62 years (range, 38–82 years) and average follow-up was 8.5 years (range, 2–16 years). Concomitant arthritic changes about the scaphoid–trapezoid joint were not a contraindication for the procedure, and the results for this subset of patients were comparable with those of the total group. Revision surgery was required in 15 of the implants. Survival of the implant was 72% at 16 years postoperatively, and the loosening rate was 44%.

Loosening was believed to be related to the constrained nature of the ball-and-socket prosthesis, with a nonphysiologic fixed center of rotation. Other factors related to loosening were altered biomechanics, the adduction deformity, and change of thumb length. The authors noted a higher rate of revision for men and younger women. The higher strain on the implant as a result of this patient population's activity level was believed to play a role in the need for revision. Not all patients with loosening were symptomatic. Half of the implants with loosening required revision particularly early out from surgery. For the other half, results were similar to those without loosening. The authors recommended the prosthesis for women, preferably older than 60 years.

The Guepar total joint arthroplasty is a cemented metal–polyethylene ball-and-socket prosthesis that is popular in France. Masmejean and colleagues[21] reported excellent or good results in all cases of 64 Guepar prostheses, with a mean follow-up of 29 months. One metacarpal stem failed, requiring removal. This second-generation prosthesis has been shown to be efficacious in providing pain relief, while improving motion and strength.[22]

The Elektra prosthesis (**Fig. 1**) is a semimodular unconstrained, cementless, hydroxyapatite-coated implant. The components are cobalt-chrome with a cup that treads into the trapezium. In his initial report of the procedure on 100 implants, Regnard,[23] who developed the prosthesis, found aseptic loosening of the trapezial cup in 15 patients, with 14 of these developing within the first 9 months. This early loosening was believed to be related to suboptimal orientation and a deficiency of bone-embedment of the trapezial cup.[24]

Ulrich-Vinther and colleagues[24] performed a prospective study comparing the Elektra prosthesis with an abductor pollicis longus tendon interposition arthroplasty. Ninety eight patients with mean age of 60 years were available for review after surgical treatment for Eaton stage II or III thumb carpometacarpal osteoarthritis. Patients with pantrapezial arthritis and poor trapezoid bone prohibiting sufficient fixation were excluded. Of the eligible patients 36 chose the cementless prosthesis and 62 underwent the tendon interposition arthroplasty. The patients were evaluated at 3, 6, and 12 months. At all postoperative visits, the patients with the Elektra prosthesis had better strength in tip pinch, key pinch, and grip. These patients also had faster and better pain relief, improved range of motion, and faster convalescence than those undergoing the tendon interposition arthroplasty. At 12 months follow-up, osteolysis was noted in two cups but no signs of implant loosening were noted. No difference was seen in complication rates. The authors noted that the cost of the prosthesis was outweighed by the socioeconomic benefits, including a more rapid recovery, earlier return to work, a minimal need for therapy, and fewer postoperative analgesics, although these parameters were not evaluated in the study.

The Braun-Cutter implant (**Fig. 2**) is a cemented articulated prosthesis with a metallic metacarpal component and polyethylene cup. The implant requires adequate trapezium height for implantation, because flattening of the trapezium or loss of height is a contraindication to the prosthesis.[15] Badia and Sambandam[15] reported good results

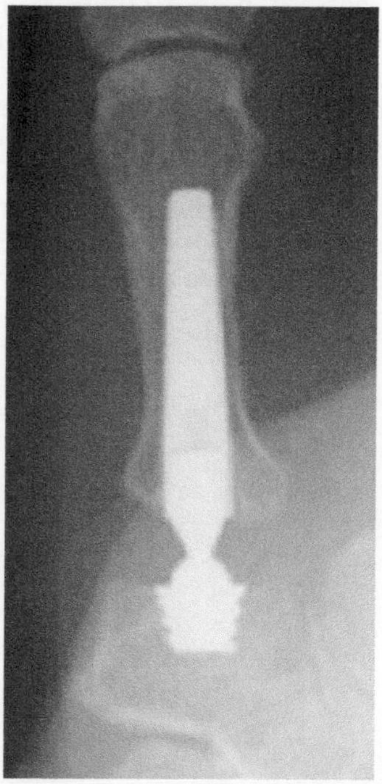

Fig. 1. Anteroposterior radiograph of an Elektra prosthesis 1 year postoperative. *From* Ulrich-Vinther M, Puggaard H, Lange B. Prospective 1-year follow-up study comparing joint prosthesis with tendon interposition arthroplasty in treatment of trapeziometacarpal osteoarthritis. J Hand Surg Am 2008;33:1372; with permission.

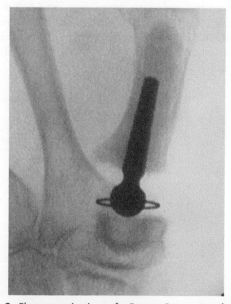

Fig. 2. Fluoroscopic view of a Braun-Cutter prosthesis. *From* Badia A, Sambandam SN. Total joint arthroplasty in the treatment of advanced stages of thumb carpometacarpal joint osteoarthritis. J Hand Surg Am 2006;31:1605.e5; with permission.

after total joint arthroplasty of the thumb carpometacarpal with this prosthesis. The series included 26 thumbs in 25 patients with an average age of 71 and average follow-up of 59 months. Indications included Eaton stage III or IV osteoarthritis. One patient had posttraumatic loosening, which required revision with satisfactory results. No radiographic signs of implant loosening were seen at final follow-up.

SURFACE REPLACEMENT

The term *surface replacement arthroplasty* has been used to describe hemiarthroplasty such as the thumb metacarpal chrome-cobalt implant or trapezial pyrolytic cup. The term also described a total surface replacement, including the articular surfaces of both the thumb metacarpal and trapezium, with implants such as the Avanta SR TMC prosthesis. These implants have been developed to limit the problem of loosening associated with total joint arthroplasty.[25]

The Avanta SR TMC prosthesis (**Fig. 3**) is a cemented total surface replacement implant consisting of two saddle-shaped components to mimic the joint contour. The thumb metacarpal articular surface is replaced with a high-density polyethylene component. The trapezium is resurfaced with a chrome-cobalt alloy with a rounded peg for anchorage in the center of the carpal bone.[25]

In a cadaveric study, Imaeda and colleagues[26] showed that resection arthroplasty and ball-and-socket joint replacements alter the normal kinematics of the thumb, thereby changing the musculotendinous moment arms and altering force transmission. Using a cadaveric model, Uchiyama and colleagues[10] showed the total joint surface replacement had similar kinematics and stability to the normal trapeziometacarpal joint, provided that a normal ligament tension was present. They found no difference in center of rotation, path of motion, or instability compared with the normal joint. The results of the study may be affected if performed on an osteoarthritic joint.

The procedure is performed through excising the proximal 3 mm of the thumb metacarpal perpendicular to the axis. The intramedullary canal is broached and the distal surface of the trapezium is removed with a bur along with any dorsal-ulnar osteophytes. A hole for the peg in the trapezium is made perpendicular to the proximal articular surface. Stability is assessed using the trial components. Both components are cemented and the dorsal capsule closed. The thumb is immobilized for 2 weeks when formalized therapy is started.

Perez-Ubeda and colleagues[27] reported poor results in 20 implants for 19 patients with an average follow-up of 33 months. They noted a 70% failure rate because of loosening among 55% of the implants and ankylosis related to periprosthetic calcification in 15%. Four patients, representing 20% of the series, required revision surgery with ligament reconstruction. A tendency toward poorer results was seen in younger patients and those with hyperextension of the metacarpophalangeal joint.

Loosening occurred in five cases despite adequate metacarpophalangeal position at insertion.[27] The increased radial slope of the trapezium implant and dorsal radial subluxation of the

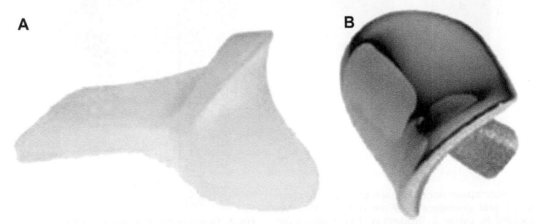

Fig. 3. The two components of the Avanta SRTM trapeziometacarpal prosthesis. (*A*) The metacarpal component composed of ultra-high molecular weight polyethylene. (*B*) The trapezial component made of cobalt chrome ally with a rounded peg for anchorage within the center of the trapezium. *From* Van Rijin J, Gosens T. A cemented surface replacement prosthesis in the basal thumb joint. J Hand Surg Am 2010;35:573; with permission.

metacarpal were found to lead to a compensatory hyperextension of the metacarpophalangeal joint. Variations in the position of the implant increased the loosening rate and radial subluxation of the metacarpal. This finding was seen in radial positioning of the trapezial implant, which was believed to be related to persistence of the medial osteophyte, underscoring the importance of complete excision of the osteophyte intraoperatively. Increased length of the thumb was also noted to be related to malposition and a poor result. Perez-Ubeda and colleagues[27] believed the malposition was related to multiple factors, and not merely the learning curve, including difficulties with the instrumentation, in contouring the distal surface of the trapezium, and in choosing the correct angle and position for the peg in the trapezium. At 2-year follow-up, 16 of the 19 patients had an excellent or good subjective functional result, although only 8 had an excellent or good result at final assessment after 3 years. The best functional results were in the more elderly patients. The authors concluded that the prosthesis was not an adequate surgical option for treating thumb carpometacarpal osteoarthritis.

Van Rijin and Gosens[25] recently reported the results of a series of 15 prostheses in 13 patients using the cemented Avanta SR TMC prosthesis. The average follow-up was 36 months. The postoperative range of motion, function with one hand, and strength did not show improvement. Significant improvement in function using both hands and decreased pain with activities occurred. No radiographic evidence of loosening was seen. One failure and one nerve injury was noted. The investigators were unable to correlate the relationship between radial position of the trapezial component, or lengthening of the trapeziometacarpal space, with poorer results described by Perez-Ubeda and colleagues.[27] The authors concluded that the Avanta SR TMC prosthesis was a reasonable surgical option for the patient with thumb carpometacarpal arthritis without involvement of the scaphoid trapezium joint.

An assessment of the literature on treatment of thumb carpometacarpal arthritis with cemented total joint arthroplasty showed major deficiencies. Sambandam and colleagues[28] analyzed the literature for methodological deficiencies and quality of outcome. Major deficiencies were noted in subject selection criteria, type of study, description of the surgical procedure, description of the rehabilitation protocol, outcomes measures, and outcomes assessment. A need exists for more prospective randomized studies with good methodology comparing cemented thumb total joint arthroplasty with other procedures.

NONAUTOLOGOUS INTERPOSITION ARTHROPLASTY

Various nonautologous materials have been used as an interpositional substance after resection arthroplasty, including silicone, polyurethaneurea, polytetrafluorethylene, acellular dermal matrix allograft, ceramic, and pyrolytic carbon.[29]

The most extensive experience with implant material for the small joints of the hand has involved silicone.[15,30] The Swanson implant has been the most commonly used silicone implant. Silicone is a rubber-like material. The common silicone elastomer was used until 1974 when the high molecular weight polymer called Silastic HP was developed to address fragmentation and collapse.[31,32] Silicone implants for the thumb carpometacarpal joint have been associated with long-term complications related to a silicone synovitis (**Fig. 4**). The shear and compression forces lead to silicone particles 15 μm or larger. The small particles of silicone are found in multinucleated giant cells as a foreign-body reaction.[33] Subluxation of the metacarpal with cystic changes also develops related to the synovitis. These changes

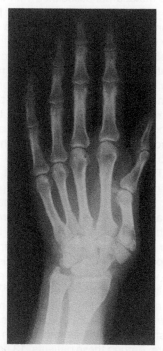

Fig. 4. Anteroposterior radiograph of the hand with radiographic evidence of a subluxated broken silicone prosthesis with silicone synovitis. *From* van Cappelle HG, Deutman R, van Horn JR. Use of the Swanson silicone trapezium implant for treatment of primary osteoarthritis. J Bone Joint Surg Am 2001;83:1000; with permission.

are noted at approximately 2 years, leading to a high failure rate.[34] Treatment options for the failed implant include removal of the prosthesis, debridement, and ligament reconstruction arthroplasty.[35]

Instability of the implant is a limitation of the procedure, with reported rates as high as 55%.[32,34,36–38] Several options have been recommended to improve stability. Swanson[32,39] suggested reinforcing the capsule with tendon slips or using a temporary Kirschner wire. Others have recommended that the osteotomy of the base of the metacarpal be made in 10° of varus to improve implant stability.[37] Eaton[40] developed an implant with a hole for tenodesis. Unfortunately, the increased stability with this implant led to increased wear, deformation, and breakage.[34]

Long-term results of the Swanson trapezium implant were reported by van Cappelle and colleagues[36] in their retrospective review of 35 patients with a mean follow-up of 13.8 years. The main complication was dislocation occurring in 18 thumbs for a rate of 40%. They believed several factors led to the instability, including the fact that the capsule was not attached to the implant on closure and because of the resultant longer lever arm of the metacarpal associated with the procedure. The authors noted that the poor long-term results confirmed their decision to stop using the implant in 1991.

The Niebauer trapeziometacarpal prosthesis is an alternative silicone implant. Dacron mesh was added for biologic fixation, and Dacron threads for fixation to prevent subluxation. The procedure is performed through removing the trapezium and the portion of the trapezoid that articulates with the scaphoid. A small amount of the base of the thumb metacarpal is removed and the canal reamed. The implant is sized so that no more than 2 mm extends beyond the margin of the scaphoid. Two holes are made in the base of the metacarpal. The Dacron threads are placed through the holes and later tied over the bone. The other two threads are placed through the flexor carpi radialis tendon. The thumb is immobilized for 6 weeks postoperatively, followed by initiation of a therapy exercise program.[30,41]

Adams and colleagues[30] performed a retrospective review of 22 Niebauer trapeziometacarpal joint arthroplasties in 18 patients with a mean follow-up of 2.4 years. Among these patients, 13 noted good pain relief, 2 were slightly improved, and 3 experienced no improvement. Asymptomatic subluxation of 50% or less occurred in 23% of the thumbs. Mechanical instability was reported in 9% of thumbs that showed greater than 75% subluxation. Implant breakage and silicone synovitis was not clinically or radiographically evident. A consistent sclerotic line was noted around the implant stem in the metacarpal, which was believed to be related to a walling off response of the bone to a foreign body. The authors noted that, despite the different design features, the study did not show better results compared with other types of silicone implants.

Sotereanos and colleagues[41] reported similar results in their retrospective review of 27 patients undergoing the Niebauer trapeziometacarpal arthroplasty with an average follow-up of 9 years. Of the patients, 88% were pleased with the result, although 83% were noted to have subluxation that increased over time. A low incidence of silicone synovitis was seen, with only one patient requiring implant removal.

In an effort to address the problem of silicone synovitis, a titanium implant for the trapeziometacarpal joint was developed. Swanson and colleagues[42] reported promising results with the implant in 1997. Putnam and Chapman[43] reported satisfactory pain relief in more than 90% of patients undergoing the procedure, with predictable and reproducible stability.

Naidu and colleagues[44] performed a finite element analysis of the titanium implant for trapeziometacarpal arthritis and predicted pistoning and maximum stress concentration at the distal tip of the prosthesis and the mid-metacarpal shaft. The clinical component of the study retrospectively reviewed 50 implants in 47 patients with an average follow-up of 2 years; 10 of the implants failed before 9 months. Implant settling occurred in varus drift and axial subsidence. The other 80% of patients showed improvements based on their disabilities of the arm, shoulder, and hand (DASH) questionnaire scores. The authors believed that the prosthesis may be suitable for low functional demand patients with good bone stock, but had stopped offering the implant to patients at their institution.

The Orthosphere (**Fig. 5**) is a spherical interposition device presented by Calandruccio and Jobe[45] in 1977. It is a simplistic approach to treating trapezoid metacarpal arthritis using an uncemented spherical interposition device made of a yttrium-stabilized zirconia.[8] Indications include stage II or III thumb carpometacarpal osteoarthritis. The implant is placed after minimal resection of the carpometacarpal joint with hemispheric reaming of both the thumb metacarpal and trapezium. The proposed advantages include a pain-free stable joint, maintaining thumb height, and not requiring tendon transfer or k-wire stabilization. The stability is obtained by the concavity created on the thumb metacarpal and trapezium. This

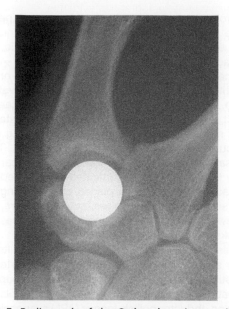

Fig. 5. Radiograph of the Orthosphere interposition arthroplasty with subsidence. *From* Athwal GS, Chenkin J, King GJ, et al. Early failures with a spheric interposition arthroplasty of the thumb basal joint. J Hand Surg Am 2004;29:1081; with permission.

implant requires limited surgical dissection, is associated with a short period of immobilization, shows low wear, and allows ease of conversion to a soft tissue interposition arthroplasty if required.[8] The early published results of the implant were promising.[45]

Athwal and colleagues[46] reported early failure in a small series of seven patients with an average follow-up of 33 months. Six of the prosthesis had subsided on follow-up. The subsidence ranged from 2 mm to complete recession into the trapezium. The proximal migration of the thumb metacarpal led to painful bone-on-bone contact. No patients were satisfied with the procedure. Five of the seven patients required revision to a resection arthroplasty with ligament reconstruction at an average of 11 months from the index surgery. No synovitis or osteolysis was noted at revision surgery. The poor short-term results led the authors to discontinue performing the procedure.

Others found good clinical results regarding pain relief, function, and patient satisfaction with the procedure, although the radiographic findings were concerning.[8] Adams and colleagues[8] performed a retrospective review of 50 implants in 49 patients with a mean 3-year follow-up. The patient satisfaction was reported as "very satisfied" or "satisfied" for 32 patients, and none were dissatisfied. Thumb pinch strength averaged 91% of the contralateral side. Most implants had

radiographic evidence of subsidence ranging from 1 to 13 mm, and 15 of the thumbs developed trapezium fractures. The authors concluded that although the mechanical aspects of the implant were attractive, the bone could not withstand the forces of the implant, leading to adverse osseous changes. Although the early clinical results were reasonable, the concern for increasing failures because of the radiographic findings caused the authors to discontinue using the implant.

Thumb carpometacarpal hemiarthroplasty has been performed with the proximal component of the Ascension MCP implant. The pyrolytic carbon prosthesis (**Fig. 6**) has an elastic modulus similar to cortical bone, which is believed to dampen stresses at the bone–prosthesis interface and improve biologic fixation.[47] Pyrolytic carbon also has been found to have good long-term biocompatibility.[48] The implant is press-fit into the thumb metacarpal canal using a technique similar to the metacarpophalangeal arthroplasty. A socket 3 to 4 mm in depth is developed in the trapezium using a small burr. If instability is noted, the depth of the cup can be increased to a level of the distal third of the trapezium. Increasing the depth of the cup further may lead to trapezium fracture. The implant is impacted into the base of the metacarpal, leaving it 2 to 3 mm proud to prevent impingement of the metacarpal base with the rim of the trapezium.

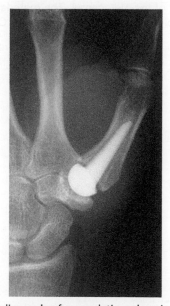

Fig. 6. Radiograph of a pyrolytic carbon implant for the thumb trapeziometacarpal joint. *From* Martinez de Aragon JS, Moran SL, Rizzo M, et al. Early outcomes of pyrolytic carbon hemiarthroplasty for the treatment of trapezial-metacarpal arthritis. J Hand Surg Am 2009;34:208; with permission.

In a retrospective review, Martinez and colleagues[47] showed mixed short-term results of the pyrolytic carbon hemiarthroplasty for the thumb carpometacarpal joint. The series included 54 joints in 49 patients, with a mean age of 59 years and a follow-up of 22 months (range, 6–54 months). All patients had Eaton stage II or III arthritis, with the diagnosis of osteoarthritis in 44 thumbs, rheumatoid arthritis in 8, psoriatic arthritis in 1, and juvenile rheumatoid arthritis in 1. Among the joints, 15 reoperations were required with 10 metacarpal subluxations, of which 7 were treated with increasing the depth of the trapezial cup.

Other techniques recommended to prevent subluxation include adequate resection of the metacarpal base, centralizing cup placement within the trapezium, use of larger implants, and strong capsular plication during wound closure. Pain relief was excellent in 35 of 49 patients, whereas 5 complained of ongoing pain without improvement. Aseptic loosening was noted in three patients. The 22-month survival rate was 80%.

The Artelon implant (**Fig. 7**) is a T-shaped prosthesis made of degradable polycaprolactone-based polyurethane urea and incorporates with the adjacent bone and connective tissue.[49,50] It acts as a spacer by providing joint separation after excision of the distal 2 mm of the trapezium, and resurfaces the joint and provides stability to the dorsal capsule.[50] The horizontal wings allow stabilization of the joint by preventing dorsal radial migration of the metacarpal. The material acts as a scaffold for tissue in-growth. Complete

hydrolysis takes approximately 6 years. Experts have proposed that with degradation, organized tissue develops and, with time, a new articular surface is formed.[50]

The procedure is performed for stage II or III arthritis. A distally based capsular flap is elevated from the proximal trapezium to the metacarpal shaft, including the dorsal capsule. The distal 1 to 2 mm of the trapezium is excised, leaving the articular surface of the metacarpal intact. The dorsal cortical surfaces of the thumb metacarpal and trapezium are decorticated to a bleeding surface. The implant is placed after soaking in saline and fixed with suture, suture anchors, or screws. The thumb is immobilized for at least 5 weeks postoperatively.

Nilsson and colleagues[50] reported the results of their series of 10 patients treated with the Artelon prosthesis and compared with a control group of 5 patients undergoing a resection arthroplasty with an abductor pollicis longus (APL) suspension. At 3 years postoperative follow-up, all patients were stable and pain-free. Range of motion was comparable between the groups. Key and chuck pinch increased from preoperative levels in the Artelon group but not the patients who had APL suspension arthroplasty. No signs were seen of foreign-body reaction.

Jorheim and colleagues[49] performed a matched cohort study with small sample size comparing the results of the Artelon implant with APL suspension arthroplasty. They concluded that the short-term results of the Artelon implant were not superior to those of the APL suspension arthroplasty. The authors evaluated the Artelon prosthesis in 13 patients with a mean age of 54 years and at a mean follow-up of 13 months. The APL suspension arthroplasty cohort consisted of 40 randomly selected patients of mean age 58 years operated on in the same period, with a follow-up of 12 months. The palmar and radial abduction was not statistically different between the groups. The QuickDASH score was 25 for the Artelon group and 20 for the patients undergoing the APL suspension arthroplasty; 8 patients undergoing the Artelon procedure were satisfied compared with 32 in the APL group. The median grip strength compared with the contralateral side was 82% and 95%, respectively. Two of the patients having an Artelon arthroplasty underwent revision to an APL arthroplasty because of persistent pain.

A foreign-body reaction can develop related to the Artelon implant.[51] Choung and Tan[52] presented a patient who developed an inflammatory reaction 12 weeks after an Artelon implant. Treatment included debridement and hematoma arthroplasty. Histology after excision showed

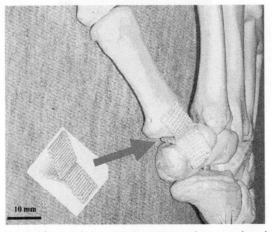

Fig. 7. The Artelon trapeziometacarpal spacer placed within the trapeziometacarpal joint. *From* Nilsson A, Liljensten E, Bergstrom C, et al. Results from a degradable TMC joint spacer (Artelon) compared with tendon arthroplasty. J Hand Surg Am 2005;30:381; with permission.

evidence of acute and chronic inflammatory changes. A second debridement was required 6 months after the resection for recurrent symptoms believed to be related to residual microfragments that remained and caused the flare. The patient had intermittent pain, and swelling at 1 year after surgery.

Other implants have also been reported to be associated with foreign-body reactions, including polytetrafluoroethylene, polypropylene, and collagen xenograft. Greenberg and colleagues[53] reported osteolytic changes adjacent to the implants in 80% of patients with a polytetrafluoroethylene (Gore-Tex) prosthesis. Muermans and Coenen[54] reported a 30% incidence of synovitis in patients with Gore-Tex implants. Belcher and Zic[55] reported adverse reactions in 6 of 13 porcine dermal collagen xenografts (Permacol). Histologic examination of 3 of the implants showed evidence of foreign-body reaction.

The Cochrane Database review[17,56,57] investigated the results of five surgical procedures of thumb arthroplasty for osteoarthritis, evaluating the results at 1 year and between 1 and 5 years. They compared trapeziectomy, trapeziectomy with interposition arthroplasty, trapeziectomy with ligament reconstruction, trapeziectomy with ligament reconstruction, and tendon interposition and joint replacement. No procedure was superior regarding pain, physical function, patient global assessment, range of motion, or strength. Trapeziectomy was noted to be safer and had fewer complications than the other procedures.

Upper-extremity surgeons continue to strive to improve the results of thumb carpometacarpal arthroplasty. The use of implants can limit the shortening of the thumb, weakness, and length of convalescence associated with resection arthroplasty. The ideal thumb carpometacarpal implant should be strong and stable, provide full range of motion, and prevent loosening. Unfortunately, no current prosthesis accomplishes all of these goals. Future implants will need to provide significant benefits that outweigh the higher costs and higher rate of revision. A larger number of well-designed prospective randomized studies will be needed to evaluate the efficacy of these procedures. Until the ideal implant is developed, clinical acumen must be used to determine appropriate patients and implants.

REFERENCES

1. Peyron JG. Osteoarthritis. The epidemiologic viewpoint. Clin Orthop Relat Res 1986;213:13–9.

2. Eaton RG, Glickel SZ. Trapeziometacarpal osteoarthritis: staging as a rationale for treatment. Hand Clin 1987;3:455–69.

3. Hartigan BJ, Stern PJ, Kiefhaber TR. Thumb carpometacarpal osteoarthritis: arthrodesis compared with ligament reconstruction and tendon interposition. J Bone Joint Surg Am 2001;83:1470–8.

4. Tomaino MM, Pellegrini VD, Burton RI. Arthroplasty of the basal joint of the thumb. Long-term follow-up after ligament reconstruction with tendon interposition. J Bone Joint Surg Am 1995;77:346–55.

5. Muller GM. Arthrodesis of the trapezio-metacarpal joint for osteoarthritis. J Bone Joint Surg Br 1949; 31:540–2.

6. Forseth MJ, Stern PJ. Complications of trapeziometacarpal arthrodesis using plate and screw fixation. J Hand Surg Am 2003;28:342–5.

7. Ishida O, Ikuta Y. Trapeziometacarpal joint arthrodesis for the treatment of arthrosis. Scand J Plast Reconstr Surg Hand Surg 2000;34:245–8.

8. Adams BD, Pomerance J, Nguyen A, et al. Early outcome of spherical ceramic trapezial-metacarpal arthroplasty. J Hand Surg Am 2009;34:213–8.

9. Cooney WP III, Chao EY. Biomechanical analysis of static forces in the thumb during hand function. J Bone Joint Surg Am 1977;59:27–36.

10. Uchiyama S, Cooney WP III, Niebur GN, et al. Biomechanical analysis of the trapexiometacarpal joint after surface replacement arthroplasty. J Hand Surg Am 1999;24:483–90.

11. Linscheid RL. Implant arthroplasty of the hand: retrospective and prospective considerations. J Hand Surg Am 2000;25:796–816.

12. Swanson AB. Silicone rubber implants for replacement of arthritis or destroyed joints in the hand. Surg Clin North Am 1968;48:1113–27.

13. Niebauer JJ, Shaw JL, Doren WW. Silicone-dacron hinge prosthesis. Design, evaluation, and application. Ann Rheum Dis 1969;28(Suppl):56–8.

14. Haffejee D. Endoprosthetic replacement of the trapezium for arthrosis in the carpometacarpal joint of the thumb. J Hand Surg Am 1977;2:141–8.

15. Badia A, Sambandam N. Total joint arthroplasty in the treatment of advanced stages of thumb carpometacarpal joint osteoarthritis. J Hand Surg Am 2006;31:1605–14.

16. Badia A. Total joint arthroplasty for the arthritic thumb carpometacarpal joint. Am J Orthop 2008; 37(8 Suppl):4–7.

17. de la Caffiniere JY, Aucouturier P. Trapeziametacarpal arthroplasty by total prosthesis. Hand 1979;11: 41–6.

18. Hamlin C. Reconstruction of the arthritic thumb carpometacarpal joint with the Caffiniere prosthesis. Atlas Hand Clin 1997;2:153–67.

19. Boeckstyns ME, Sinding A, Elholm KT, et al. Replacement of the trapeziometacarpal joint with

a cemented (Caffiniere) prosthesis. J Hand Surg Am 1989;14:83–9.

20. van Cappelle HG, Elzenga P, van Horn JR. Long-term results and loosening analysis of de la Caffiniere replacements of the trapeziometacarpal joint. J Hand Surg Am 1999;24:476–82.

21. Masmejean E, Alnot JY, Chantelot C, et al. Guepar anatomical trapeziometacarpal prosthesis. Chir Main 2003;22:30–6.

22. Lemoine S, Wavreille G, Alnot JY, et al. Second generation GUEPAR total arthroplasty of the thumb basal joint: 50 months follow-up in 84 cases. Orthop Traumatol Surg Res 2009;95:63–9.

23. Regnard PJ. Electra trapeziometacarpal prosthesis: results of the first 100 cases. J Hand Surg Br 2006; 31:621–8.

24. Ulrich-Vinther M, Puggaard H, Lange B. Prospective 1-year follow-up study comparing joint prosthesis with tendon interposition arthroplasty in treatment of trapeziometacarpal osteoarthritis. J Hand Surg Am 2008;33:1360–77.

25. Van Rijin J, Gosens T. A cemented surface replacement prosthesis in the basal thumb joint. J Hand Surg Am 2010;35:572–9.

26. Imaeda T, An KN, Cooney WP, et al. Kinematics of the trapeziometacarpal joint: a biomechanical analysis comparing tendon interposition arthroplasty and total joint arthroplasty. J Hand Surg Am 1996; 21:544–53.

27. Perez-Ubeda MJ, Garcia-Lopez A, Martinez FM, et al. Results of the cemented SR trapexiometacarpal prosthesis in the treatment of thumb carpometacarpal osteoarthritis. J Hand Surg Am 2003;28: 917–25.

28. Sambandam SN, Gul A, Priyanka P. Analysis of methodological deficiencies of studies reporting surgical outcome following cemented total-joint arthroplasty of trapezio-metacarpal joint of the thumb. Int Orthop 2007;31:630–45.

29. Forthman CL. Management of advanced trapexiometacarpal arthrosis. J Hand Surg Am 2009;34: 331–4.

30. Adams BD, Unsell RS, McLaughlin P. Niebauer trapeziometacarpal arthroplasty. J Hand Surg Am 1990;15:487–92.

31. Ruffin RA, Rayan GM. Treatment of trapeziometacarpal arthritis with silastic and metallic implant arthroplasty. Hand Clin 2001;17:245–53.

32. Swanson AB, deGoot Swanson G, Watermen JJ. Trapezium implant arthroplasty: long-term evaluation of 150 cases. J Hand Surg Am 1981;6:125–41.

33. Karlsson MK, Necking LE, Redlund-Johnell I. Foreign body reaction after modified silicone rubber arthroplasty of the first carpometacarpal joint. Scand J Plast Reconstr Surg 1992;26:101–3.

34. Pellegrini VD, Burton RI. Surgical management of basal joint arthritis of the thumb. Part I. Long-term

results of silicone implant arthroplasty. J Hand Surg Am 1986;11:309–24.

35. Van Heest AE, Kallemeier P. Thumb carpal metacarpal arthritis. J Am Acad Orthop Surg 2008;16: 140–51.

36. van Cappelle HG, Deutman R, Horn JR. Use of the Swanson silicone trapezium implant for treatment of primary osteoarthritis. J Bone Joint Surg Am 2001;83:999–1004.

37. Allieu Y, Pequignot JP, Asencio G, et al. Swanson trapezial implant in the treatment of peritrapezial arthrosis. A study of eighty cases. Ann Chir Main 1984;3:113–23.

38. Peimer CA. Long-term complications of trapeziometacarpal silicone arthroplasty. Clin Orthop Relat Res 1987;220:86–9.

39. Swanson AB. Disabling arthritis at the base of the thumb: treatment by resection of the trapeziumand flexible (silicone) implant arthroplasty. J Bone Joint Surg Am 1972;54:456–71.

40. Eaton RG. Replacement of the trapezium for arthritis of the basal articulations: a new technique with stabilization by tenodesis. J Bone Joint Surg Am 1979;61:76–82.

41. Sotereanos DG, Taras J, Urbaniak JR. Niebauer trapeziometacarpal arthroplasty: a long-term follow-up. J Hand Surg Am 1993;18:560–4.

42. Swanson AB, deGroot Swanson G, DeHeer DH, et al. Carpal bone titanium implant arthroplasty. 10 years' experience. Clin Orthop Relat Res 1997; 342:46–58.

43. Putnam M, Chapman J. Interpositional titanium hemiarthroplasty for trapezial metacarpal arthritis. Atlas Hand Clin 1997;2:203–16.

44. Naidu SH, Kulkarni N, Saunders M. Titanium basal joint arthroplasty: a finite element analysis and clinical study. J Hand Surg Am 2006;31: 760–5.

45. Calandruccio J, Jobe M. Arthroplasty of the thumb carpometacarpal joint. Semin Arthroplasty 1997;8: 135–47.

46. Athwal GS, Chenkin J, King GJ, et al. Early failures with a spheric interposition arthroplasty of the thumb basal joint. J Hand Surg Am 2004;29:1080–4.

47. Martinez de Aragon JS, Moran SL, Rizzo M, et al. Early outcomes of pyrolytic carbon hemiarthroplasty for the treatment of trapezial-metacarpal arthritis. J Hand Surg Am 2009;34:205–12.

48. Cook SD, Beckenbaugh RD, Redondo J, et al. Long-term follow-up of pyrolytic carbon metacarpophalangeal implants. J Bone Joint Surg Am 1999; 81:635–48.

49. Jorheim M, Isaxon I, Flondell M, et al. Short-term outcomes of trapeziometacarpal Artelon implant compared with tendon suspension interposition arthroplasty for osteoarthritis: a matched cohort study. J Hand Surg Am 2009;34:1381–7.

50. Nilsson A, Liljensten E, Bergstrom C, et al. Results from a degradable TMC joint spacer (Artelon) compared with tendon arthroplasty. J Hand Surg Am 2005;30:380–9.

51. Giuffrida AY, Gyuricza C, Perino G, et al. Foreign body reaction to Artelon spacer: case report. J Hand Surg Am 2009;34:1388–92.

52. Choung EW, Tan V. Foreign-body reaction to the Artelon CMC joint spacer: case report. J Hand Surg Am 2008;33:1617–20.

53. Greenberg JA, Mosher JF, Fatti JF. X-ray changes after expanded polytetrafluoroethylene (Gor-Tex) interpositional arthroplasty. J Hand Surg Am 1997;22:658–63.

54. Muermans S, Coenen L. Interpositional arthroplasty with Gore-Tex, Marlex or tendon for osteoarthritis of the trapeziometacarpal joint. A retrospective comparative study. J Hand Surg Br 1998;23:64–8.

55. Belcher HJ, Zic R. Adverse effect of porcine collagen interposition after trapeziectomy: a comparative study. J Hand Surg Br 2001;26:159–64.

56. Wajon A, Edmunds AL. Surgery for thumb (trapeziometacarpal joint) osteoarthritis. Cochrane Database Syst Rev 2009;4:CD004631.

57. Sai S, Fujii K, Chino J, et al. Tendon suspension sling arthroplasty for degenerative arthritis of the thumb trapeziometacarpal joint: long-term follow-up. J Orthop Sci 2004;9:576–80.

Interposition Arthroplasty Options for Carpometacarpal Arthritis of the Thumb

Nathan D. Bodin, MD, MS[a], Ryan Spangler, BS[b], Joseph J. Thoder, MD[a],*

KEYWORDS

- Carpometacarpal arthritis • Suspensionplasty
- Interposition arthroplasty • Arthroplasty
- Ligament reconstruction

Surgical treatment of carpometacarpal (CMC) arthritis of the thumb, or basal joint arthritis, has been and continues to be an evolving solution. As the second most common location for osteoarthritis in the upper limb after the distal interphalangeal joints[1,2] the prevalence of CMC arthritis of the thumb and its potentially painful sequelae has led this pathology to be the focus of much research and innovation. This article reviews historical surgical solutions and addresses options in ligament reconstruction and interposition arthroplasty, including the authors' preferred method.

Although postmenopausal women are the most common thumb CMC arthritis patients,[3] with 40% to 57% exhibiting radiographic evidence of disease,[4,5] other populations, including middle-aged women and men over 75 years of age, have significant joint involvement at 10% and 25%, respectively.[4] Thumb CMC arthritis is a potentially debilitating condition causing pain and weakness with the essential movements of the first metacarpal-trapezial joint: opposition, key pinch (prehension), and circumduction. Pain is localized to the base of the thumb but may radiate proximally to the radial forearm. The synovitis and effusion of early disease[1] may be associated with thenar tenderness and first webspace cramping.[6] As the disease progresses, associated subjective instability and objective deformity are noted as the shoulder sign, or the radial prominence of the dorsally subluxed first metacarpal. Classic findings of crepitence with motion of the arthritic joint, pain with a dorsal shearing force on the base of the subluxed metacarpal, and a positive grind test, or longitudinal compression of the first ray in a circular motion, may be noted. Eaton and Littler[1] described a pathognomonic finding for early disease by eliciting pain with distraction of a slightly flexed first ray with axial rotation.

Radiographic diagnosis is made based on standard views, including the Roberts CMC view (**Fig. 1**) and a pronated, anteroposterior radiographic view centered on the thumb CMC joint as well as lateral and the oblique stress view (**Fig. 2**) taken posteroanterior with the patient's thumbs pressed together at their radial borders. Staging is made according to the classification established by Eaton and Littler in 1973, modified in 1987 by Eaton and Glickel.[7] It is based on bony changes, joint subluxation, and osteophyte formation (**Table 1**). Eaton stage I has subtle radiographic changes, including widening of the joint space secondary to synovitis and effusion, but the CMC joint remains well reduced. Stage II begins to show classic arthritic changes with joint space narrowing and sclerosis. Osteophytes are less than 2 mm and joint subluxation is less than one-third the width of the metacarpal base. In

[a] Department of Orthopaedic Surgery and Sports Medicine, Temple University Hospital, Outpatient Building, 6th Floor, 3401 North Broad Street, Philadelphia, PA 19140, USA
[b] Temple University School of Medicine, 3500 North Broad Street, Philadelphia, PA 19140, USA
* Corresponding author.
E-mail address: Joseph.thoder@tuhs.temple.edu

Hand Clin 26 (2010) 339–350
doi:10.1016/j.hcl.2010.05.006

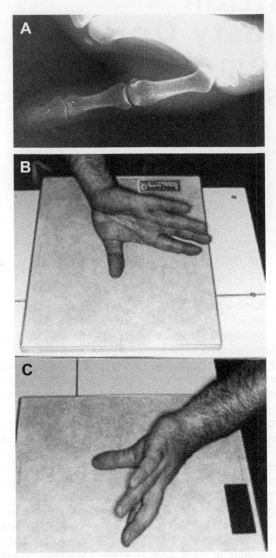

Fig. 1. Roberts view: (*A*) anteroposterior view of thumb CMC joint and (*B*) dorsal and (*C*) volar photos of positioning for radiograph. (*From* Special X ray views of the thumb. In: E-hand.com the electronic textbook of hand surgery. 2009. Available at: http://www.eatonhand.com/ray/ray012.htm; with permission.)

stage III, a narrow, sclerotic joint is seen along with the presence of large osteophytes and joint subluxation greater than 33%. Stage IV has been revised to describe pantrapezial arthritis—disease encompassing all four joints: trapeziometacarpal, scaphotrapezial, trapezium-index metacarpal, and trapezium-trapezoid. The significance of this staging system becomes clear as the biomechanical and pathophysiologic relationships of the principal CMC joint complex ligaments and the deforming forces acting on it are considered.

ANATOMY AND PATHOPHYSIOLOGY

The diarthrodial saddle joint of the first metacarpal-trapezial joint allows anatomic range of motion in two orthogonal planes: flexion-extension and abduction-adduction. As the joint is relatively unconstrained, a third rotary motion is permitted by the saddles twisting relative to one and other. The sleeve of ligamentous support for this joint is tensioned by this twisting moment, which adds extrinsic stability to the trapeziometacarpal joint in circumduction and opposition.[1] Of the 16 ligaments identified, the deep anterior oblique ligament, or beak ligament, and the dorsal radial ligament have been shown to be the principal checkreins to dorsal subluxation during physiologic motion of the joint.[8]

The deep anterior oblique ligament is intra-articular and courses from the beak, or volar tip, of the metacarpal saddle to the volar articular

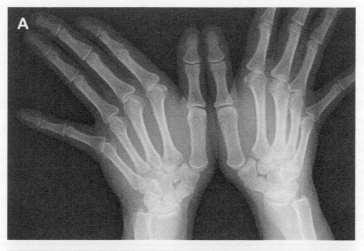

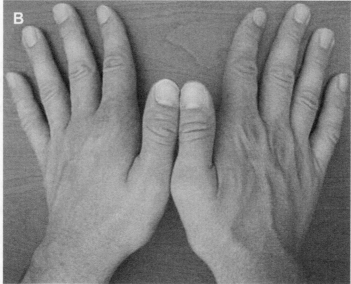

Fig. 2. (*A*) Bilateral thumb CMC stress view: posteroanterior oblique radiographic view (*above*) and (*B*) photo of patient pushing radial border of bilateral thumbs together (*below*). (*From* Special X ray views of the thumb. In: E-hand.com the electronic textbook of hand surgery. 2009. Available at: http://www.eatonhand.com/ray/ray012. htm; with permission.)

border of the trapezium. It is located at the pivot point for opposition and is thus tight in most motions, preventing dorsal subluxation of the metacarpal during pinch. The dorsal radial ligament is a broad capsular thickening oriented longitudinally opposite and radial to the deep anterior oblique ligament. It is tight in supination and functions as the second most important stabilizer preventing dorsal subluxation during grip and pinch.[8]

During motions, such as key pinch, the incongruity of the articular surfaces causes apex loading on the volar articular surface of the trapezium, transmitting loads of up to 13 times the joint reactive force.[8] With repeated eccentric wear,

osteoarthitic changes begin volarly in CMC disease. Any laxity or incompetence to the anterior oblique ligament allows this fulcrum to move dorsally and adds to the eccentric force concentration, propagating arthritic change dorsally with subluxation.[1,9] Concomitantly, the biochemical milieu of arthritis creates a hostile environment for the chondral surface and contributes to degenerative change.[9]

TREATMENT OPTIONS

Three principles based on the core pathology of CMC arthritis dictate all of the treatment options discussed: (1) removal of diseased joint surfaces,

---

Table 1
Eaton and Glickel's radiographic classification system of CMC arthritis of the thumb

Staging	Radiographic Characteristics
Stage I	Normal or slightly widened trapeziometacarpal joint Normal articular contours Trapeziometacarpal subluxation (if present up to one-third of the articular surface)
Stage II	Decreased trapeziometacarpal joint space Trapeziometacarpal subluxation (if present up to one-third of the articular surface) Osteophytes or loose bodies less than 2 mm in diameter
Stage III	Further decrease in trapeziometacarpal joint space Subchondral cysts or sclerosis Osteophytes or loose bodies 2 mm or more in diameter Trapeziometacarpal joint subluxation of one-third or more of the articular surface
Stage IV	Involvement of the scaphotrapezial joint or less commonly the trapeziotrapezoid or trapeziometacarpal joint to the index finger

Adapted from Matullo KS, Ilyas A, Thoder JJ. CMC arthroplasty of the thumb: a review. Hand (N Y) 2007;2(4):232–9; with permission.

---

(2) reconstruction of ligamentous stabilizers, and (3) preservation of the arthroplasty space.[10,11] The third concept represents the broad notion of preventing secondary morbidity—from impingement or subsidence of the new joint surfaces, donor site morbidity from autologous tendon harvests, or introduction of immunogenic materials that may cause reactions, for example. Early procedures that failed to address all three considerations have been shown to provide less durable or satisfactory results compared with modern techniques.

Ligament Reconstruction with Tendon Interposition Arthroplasty

The most frequently used surgical solution for Eaton stage II-IV CMC arthritis is the trapeziectomy and ligament reconstruction with or without tendon interposition arthroplasty; however, LRTI is not a single procedure but a menu of separate surgical options—each with a relevant history and currently recommended treatment. The common surgical goal for these three procedures is to provide strong, durable, pain-free range of motion in CMC joint of the thumb while still fulfilling the three core principalse.

History: LRTI

Early surgical treatment of painful CMC arthritis was total trapeziectomy, first described in 1949 by Gervis[12] with satisfactory relief of pain; however, subsequent studies, including a long-term retrospective case review by Gervis and Wells,[13] demonstrated troublesome weakness and instability. Without the ligamentous support of the trapeziometacarpal ligaments and the

structural support of the intact radial column of the wrist, metacarpal subsidence into the arthroplasty space changes the mechanical relationship of the thumb in pinch and grip and contributed to the subjective failure of simple trapeziectomy.

Kuhns and colleagues[14] addressed the problem of proximal migration of the metacarpal into the trapezium space by temporarily holding the metacarpal in a slightly distracted position by Kirschner (K)-wire fixation to the index metacarpal. After 6 to 8 weeks in a spica cast, pins are removed and range of motion begun. In their series of 26 patients treated in this manner, complete resolution of symptoms was reported by 74% at 6 months and 92% at 2-year follow-up. Grip, key, and tip-pinch strength improved by 47%, 33%, and 22%, respectively, at 2 years. Proximal migration of the metacarpal into the trapezial space averaged 60% on 2-year follow-up stress radiographs.[14]

The seminal article surgically addressing the etiology of ligamentous instability is the Eaton and Littler[1] 1973 article introducing ligament reconstruction for the painful thumb CMC joint. They identified the volar beak ligament, also known as the deep volar anterior oblique ligament, as the principal checkrein to dorsal subluxation of the thumb metacarpa. They proposed to redirect the radial portion of the flexor carpi radialis (FCR) tendon through a sagital bone tunnel at the base of the thumb metacarpal to reconstruct the ligament—anatomically and biomechanically. In their technique, visible osteophytes are excised on CMC joint inspection but no trapeziectomy is performed.

In their initial series of 18 patients with stage II to IV CMC treated with their ligament reconstruction, Eaton and Littler reported 100% of stage II patients had excellent results: no pain, postoperative grip strength within 10% of the nonoperative hand, and no further radiographic changes at follow-up of at least 1 year. Stage III patients demonstrated 63% excellent and 37% good results: occasional pain with pinch, strength less than 90% of nonoperative side, and minor radiographic deterioration. Patients with stage IV disease scored 60% good or excellent and 40% fair results: pain with regular use and joint deterioration at or worse than preoperative state.[1]

The reported pain and deterioration after ligament reconstruction without trapeziectomy for patients with stage IV—pantrapezial—disease underscores the importance of resection of the painful, arthritic joint surfaces. In a subsequent 1985 series by Eaton and coworkers[15] evaluating FCR-ligament reconstruction for stage III disease only, 92% good or excellent results were reported. The improvement from their prior study is attributed to the creation of a small arthroplasty space by resection of the metacarpal base, planing of the trapezium, and FCR tendon interposition to prevent further arthritic change.

The method of Burton and Pellegrini[10] introduced the concept of ligament reconstruction interposition arthroplasty (LRTI). The durability of their technique (described later) has been proved by a long-term follow-up. The authors use a partial thickness FCR autograft to reconstruct the volar oblique ligament in a variation of the Eaton and Littler technique. In addition, an FCR tendon interposition mass, or anchovy, is used to stabilize the arthroplasty space,[10] based on Froimson's original description.[16]

In a retrospective series of 25 thumbs treated with LRTI and hemitrapeziectomy (stage II and III), or complete trapeziectomy (stage IV, pantrapezial disease) followed for an average of 2 years postoperatively, 92% reported excellent pain relief and an aggregate 19% increase in pinch and grip strength compared with preoperative measurements. Radiographs demonstrated a 7% dynamic subluxation and 11% proximal migration of the metacarpal. All patients returned to work and subjects included machine operators, drivers, and concert pianists. Complications included 2 reports of paresthesias in the palmar sensory branch of the median nerve and 1 report of transient reflex sympathetic dystrophy.[10]

Long-term follow-up of this series was continued and evaluation reported at 6 and 9 years. Ninety-two percent of patients were satisfied with their pain relief and activity at 9 years

follow-up. Strength measurements continued to improve: grip and tip pinch improved by 93% and 65%, respectively, compared with preoperative values, but the greatest gains were made in the first 6 years. Key pinch improvements were noted between the 2-year and 6-year intervals but decreased at final follow-up, although there was still a 34% improvement overall versus preoperative values. Radiographically, metacarpal dynamic subluxation was measured at 11% and proximal migration was 13% at 9 years[11]—a minimal degeneration compared with postoperative values of 7% subluxation and 11% proximal migration.[10] The durable results of the LRTI in the hands of these investigators merit careful study of their technique.

Technique: LRTI

A volar-radial triradiate incision centered over the trapezium is used for exposure of the trapeziometacarpal joint. Alternatively, a dorsoradial oblique or straight radial approach between the glaborous and nonglaborous skin incision may be used. After identification and protection of the nerve and artery, the capsule over the trapezium is opened longitudinally and the edges are tagged. All joints are inspected. Using an oscillating saw, the articular surface of the thumb metacarpal is removed, proximal to the insertion of the abductor pollicis brevis. A complete trapeziectomy is routinely performed and removed piecemeal leaving the intact FCR tendon. An oblique bony tunnel is made with a power burr from the volar aspect of the cut base of the metacarpal through the dorsal cortex distally and widened with gouges to approximately 6 mm diameter.

In a modification from the originally described technique, the entire width of the FCR can be harvested at the musculotendinous junction and brought into the trapeziectomy space via several transverse incisions in the volar forearm. These investigators[11] repair any capsular rents and place a tag suture in the volar capsule to affix the interposition mass at a later point. After mobilizing the FCR to its insertion the free end of the tendon is retrieved with a 30-gauge wire through the first metacarpal bony tunnel: tendon in at the base and out of the dorsal cortex.

The construct is tensioned by first distracting the thumb until the base is level with that of the index metacarpal and oriented as in a fist position. A 0.045-inch K-wire is used to percutaneously fix the metacarpal to the ulnar carpus, taking care not to violate the bony tunnel or prevent tendon sliding during tensioning. Once fixed, the slack is taken out of the FCR at the insertion and pulled tightly through the tunnel where it is sutured to the dorsal periosteum. The tendon is then folded over the cut metacarpal base and sutured to itself, thus resurfacing the metacarpal.

The remaining tendon is fashioned into the anchovy by folding itself over four times and skewering the mass with two parallel Keith needles. Each corner of the stack is sutured. The previously placed volar capsular tag suture is threaded—one limb through each Keith needle—and the whole interposition mass snugged into the trapeziectomy space creating an insertional arthroplasty. The extensor pollicis brevis is tenodesed to the metacarpal shaft proximal to the metacarpalphalangeal joint "to eliminate the hyperextension moment acting on the proximal phalanx."

The capsule is tightly closed in two layers followed by skin closure and immobilization in a long-arm spica cast for 4 weeks. At follow-up, the cast and K-wire are removed and range-of-motion exercises are started in a removable thumb spica splint. Resisted strengthening is started at 3 months after postoperative radiographs and discontinuation of the splint. Full activity is anticipated at 4 to 6 months postoperatively.[11]

Outcome: LRTI

The Burton and Pellegrini LRTI or variations thereof have been the mainstay of current treatment for advanced thumb CMC arthritis but as the procedure is dissected into it constituent parts, there has been a torrent of clinical research aimed at determining the optimal combination of ligament reconstruction options, necessity of interposition mass, and benefits of trapeziectomy.

The issue of whether or not the trapeziectomy is necessary has been largely laid to rest in light of the durability, pain control, and radiographic stability of the series[10,11]; however, in younger patients for which a salvage arthrodesis is an important future option, hemitrapeziectomy may preserve vital bone stock.[11]

After a trapeziectomy, maintenance of the arthroplasy space has been addressed (discussed previously) by interposition mass, K-wire fixation, ligament reconstruction, or any combination of the three. A report by Froimson[16] and study by Menon and colleagues[17] describe pain and proximal migration of the metacarpal at follow-up after trapeziectomy with ligament interposition only. The question of the necessity of an interposition mass in the context of ligament reconstruction has been raised and there are several series in which positive results without interposition suggest that this intervention is not necessary.[18–21]

This assertion was directly tested in a prospective, randomized study by Gerwin and colleagues[20] comparing trapeziectomy with LRTI.

Group one received a tendon interposition in the method of Burton and Pellegrini but without K-wire fixation. Group II underwent a first metacarpal suspension using with one-half of the FCR tendon harvested locally within the volar wrist incision and fixed with a suture anchor to the metacarpal but without tendon interposition. No difference was noted between the two groups with respect to grip and pinch strength, functional testing, or satisfaction. Radiographic evaluation of proximal migration also showed no significant difference between LRTI.[20]

These findings were echoed by Kriegs-Au and colleagues[18] in a prospective, randomized clinical trial of 43 patients (52 thumbs) undergoing complete trapeziectomy with LRTI. Comparisons between the treatment groups were made based on pain, daily function, strength, and radiographic proximal migration of the thumb metacarpal at 4 years. No statistically significant difference was demonstrated between the group with interposition arthroplasty and the group without.[18]

Investigating potential morbidity at donor tendons, Naidu and colleagues[22] compared biomechanical parameters of flexion and extension torque and fatigue strength in addition to grip and pinch strength and disabilities of the arm, shoulder, and hand (DASH) scores between thumbs treated with trapeziectomy and LRTI. The graft material used was entire-width FCR tendon. The nonoperative, contralateral thumb was used as a control. Postoperatively, all patients were followed for a minimum of 24 months. In this study, DASH scores improved from 43 to 12, and grip and pinch strength significantly improved. The contralateral extremity had 2.5 times more fatigue resistance with flexion resistance, and the flexion/extension torque ratio decreased on the operative side.[22–26]

Interposition Arthroplasty

Silicone implants have been used as interposition devices after trapeziectomy[27] and in resurfacing—hemiarthroplasy—procedures[28] to address late-stage CMC arthritis. In long-term follow-up and head-to-head comparison with trapeziectomy-LRTI, silicone implants have been shown to cause synovitis, pain, and high rate of revision.[27,29] Total joints and implant arthroplasty, however, are outside the scope of this discussion.

Alternatively, Gore-Tex (W.L. Gore & Associates, Newark, DE, USA) and Marlex (Chevron Phillips, Houston, TX, USA) synthetic polymers have been used as interposition materials after trapeziectomy. Greenberg and colleagues[30] used a folded Gore-Tex interposition mass in 34 thumbs after

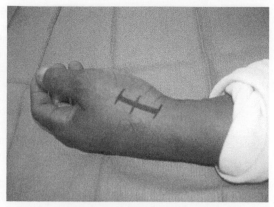

Fig. 3. Skin incision along first dorsal compartment centered over the trapezium.

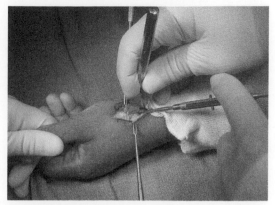

Fig. 5. The trapezium is divided in cruciate fashion with a small, straight osteotome.

trapeziectomy for advanced CMC arthritis. Radiographic evidence of osteolysis was present in 80% of cases, mostly in the proximal first metacarpal and distal pole of the scaphoid. As in most other studies, postoperative grip and pinch strength improved. Histologic analysis of osteolytic bone at time of revision showed giant cells, denoting a reactive process secondary to particulate matter.[30] A study comparing Marlex, Gore-Tex, and FCR tendon interposition without ligament reconstruction mirrored these findings in the Gore-Tex group with particulate synovitis and osteolysis requiring revision. The Marlex group had a 44% complication rate and required one revision procedure. The authors have discontinued the use of Gore-Tex interposition in their patients.[31] Similarly, Marlex was considered to be a poor replacement to autologous tendon interposition given the rate of complications. Porcine dermal xenograft

likewise resulted in failure secondary to immunogenicity.[32]

A newer alternative interposition arthroplasty option is acellular dermal matrix allograft. Graft-Jacket (Wright Medical Technology, Arlington, TN, USA) is a biologic collagen scaffold made from donated cadaveric dermis treated by a proprietary method to remove cellular elements, thus rendering it, theoretically, nonimmunogenic while preserving its biomechanical strength characteristics.[33] It has been used successfully as an allograft augmentation in Achilles tendon and rotator cuff repairs[34–36] and recently as an arthroscopic interposition mass in glenoid resurfacing and post-trapeziectomy in CMC arthritis.[37,38]

Preclinical models demonstrated full biologic incorporation and vascularization within 2 weeks in an athymic rat and no inflammatory or immunologic response against the graft after bony healing

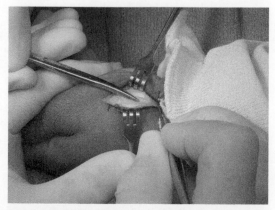

Fig. 4. The first dorsal compartment is entered between abductor pollicis longus and extensor pollicis brevis while the radial artery and superficial branch of the radial nerve are gently retracted.

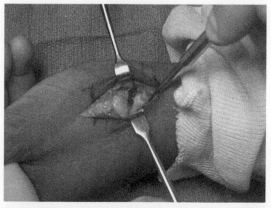

Fig. 6. The intact FCR tendon and surfaces of first metacarpal, scaphoid, trapezoid, and index metacarpal are inspected.

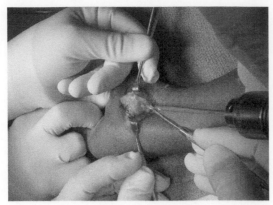

Fig. 7. Drilling of the intermedullary canal from articular surface along the long axis of the thumb metacarpal.

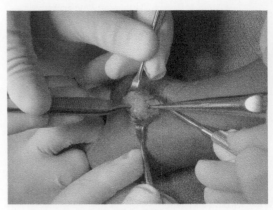

Fig. 9. Two curettes or small instruments are used to widen tunnels until they "spoon" at the junction.

in a porcine bone defect–bridging study.[33] In a canine full-thickness rotator cuff tear model, GraftJacket was compared with autologous tendon graft and found to have equal strength profiles at 12 weeks. Histologic appearance of allograft was identical to that of native tendon at 6 months.[39] According to clinical and preclinical data, acellular dermal allograft seems a possible alternative graft material that has biomechanical properties similar to autologous tendon grafts and is not immunogenic.

LIGAMENT RECONSTRUCTION WITH ACELLULAR DERMAL MATRIX ALLOGRAFT

Ligament reconstruction arthroplasty using acellular dermal matrix allograft is a new development in the surgical management of CMC arthritis. This procedure addresses the treatment principles for CMC arthritis with the potential benefits of decreased operative time[40] while eliminating possible donor site morbidity and wrist flexion weakness from autologous FCR tendon harvest. It has become the treatment of choice at the authors' institution and at others.

In a retrospective case series, Kokkalis and colleagues[41] performed a complete trapeziectomy with ligament reconstruction and interposition arthroplasty using the acellular dermal matrix allograft, GraftJacket, on 82 thumbs with stage II to IV CMC arthritis. No autologous tendon graft was harvested in any of their cases. Patients were followed for an average of 30 months. Postoperatively they were able to demonstrate significantly reduced pain scores from 6.2 to 0.7 and improvements in grip and key pinch strength by 16% and 19%, respectively. Assessment of the arthroplasty space on postoperative posteroanterior and oblique nonstress radiographs demonstrated an average of 33% metacarpal subsidence at follow-up with no signs of degenerative changes or metacarpal-scaphoid impingement.

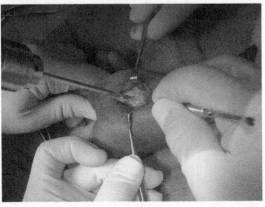

Fig. 8. Drilling of the dorsal cortex of the thumb perpendicular to the thumbnail.

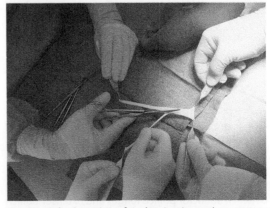

Fig. 10. Rehydrated GraftJacket is trimmed to approximately 7 mm width.

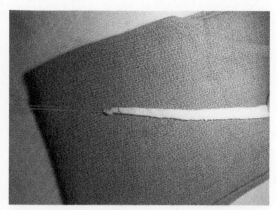

Fig. 11. Modified Kessler stitch through tapered, leading end of graft.

The investigators noted no complications or reactions to the acellular dermal allograf but reported two revision surgeries for pain or instability, although they stated that these were likely due to premorbid conditions and decidedly not secondary to use of allograft.[41]

Technique: Ligament Reconstruction and Suspensionplasty with Acellular Dermal Allograft

The use of the acellular dermal matrix allograft, GraftJacket, for ligament reconstruction and suspensionplasty has been the authors' preferred technique since 2006 for stage II-IV CMC arthritis. At time of surgical consent, it is explained to patients at length that the use of the allograft for this procedure is an off-label use.

A 4-cm skin incision is made along the first dorsal compartment centered at the trapezium (**Fig. 3**). Dissection continues to the first dorsal compartment, identifying and protecting branches of the superficial radial nerve and artery. Superficial veins and small arterial branches are coagulated with bipolar cautery. The first compartment is entered between the abductor pollicis longus and extensor pollicis brevis (**Fig. 4**), which are retracted gently with a retractor exposing the capsule. Using a #64 blade, the capsule is incised longitudinally from the proximal first metacarpal to the scaphotrapezial joint.

The capsule is sharply dissected from the trapezium and proximal metacarpal in a full-thickness flap. Using a small osteotome, the trapezium is divided in cruciate fashion and removed piecemeal (**Fig. 5**). The joint surfaces and intact FCR tendon insertion are inspected (**Fig. 6**). A small rongeur is used to remove osteophytes from the base of the first metacarpal if necessary.

A standard 3-mm drill bit is used to enter the intermedullary canal of the first metacarpal from the center of the articular surface to a depth of 5 to 7 mm parallel to the axis of the shaft (**Fig. 7**). A second drill hole is made in the dorsal cortex 5 mm distal to the end of the articular cartilage perpendicular to the nail bed to meet the first drill hole (**Fig. 8**). Two small, straight curettes are used to widen and smooth the bony tunnels at the junction of the two drill holes to ensure a patent and uniform tunnel (**Fig. 9**).

On the back table, the GraftJacket acellular dermal allograft is rehydrated in sterile saline according the manufacturer's specifications. Dr Joseph Thoder prefers the 1 × 12–cm GraftJacket Maxstrip. The strip is grasped at all four corners with forceps and trimmed to a width of approximately 7 mm with the leading edge tapered (**Fig. 10**). A 3-0 Ethibond (Ethicon, Mexico City, Mexico) modified Kessler stitch is placed in the

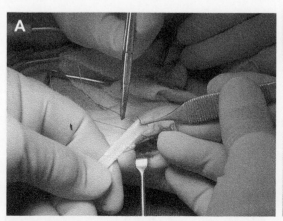
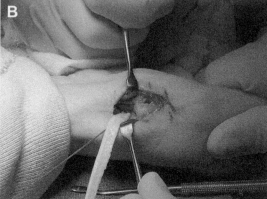

Fig. 12. (*A*) Horizontal suture in graft. (*B*) Graft sutured end-to-side to FCR. Trailing end of graft is sutured end to side to FCR.

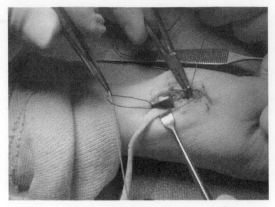

Fig. 13. Thin wire loop is used to pass graft antero-grade through the bony tunnel.

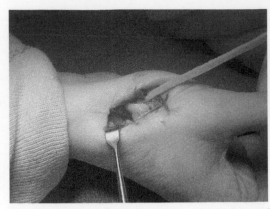

Fig. 15. Tensioning of the graft with thumb abducted and distracted.

leading edge to assist in drawing the graft through the metacarpal tunnel (**Fig. 11**). The graft is then brought into the field.

Using 3-0 Ethibond sutures, the broad end of the GraftJacket is sutured end to side to the FCR just proximal to its insertion on the second meta-carpal (**Fig. 12**). A thin wire loop is passed retro-grade from dorsal to articular through the bony tunnel (**Fig. 13**) and used to retrieve the leading edge suture from the tapered end of the graft, which is drawn through the tunnel to exit the dorsal cortex (**Fig. 14**), thus reconstructing the volar obli-que ligament. With the thumb abducted, the graft is tensioned to suspend the first metacarpal in the appropriate position (**Fig. 15**), taking care to avoid impingement of the first metacarpal base on the index metacarpal or the trapezoid. The re-maining graft is looped back behind itself, deep to the graft entering the metacarpal base, and sutured back to the intact FCR tendon (**Fig. 16**). No interposition mass is created.

The arthroplasty space is irrigated and the capsule snugly closed with 2-0 vicryl sutures or imbricated if preoperatively stretched by the sub-luxing metacarpal. Skin is closed with 5-0 nylon in-terrupted sutures and sterilely dressed and a thumb spica splint placed. At 2 weeks, sutures are removed and a removable, short-arm spica splint is placed for 4 weeks during which gentle active range of motion is started. Strengthening and activities of daily living are begun at 6 weeks, progressing to no restrictions by approximately 3 months.

Outcome: Acellular Dermal Allograft

The authors have retrospectively reviewed their experience with the use of the acellular dermal allograft ligament reconstruction and tendon inter-position for thumb CMC arthritis in comparison with their prior technique of traditional split-FCR LRTI.

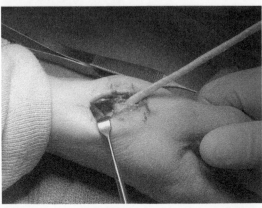

Fig. 14. The graft is drawn anterograde through the tunnel.

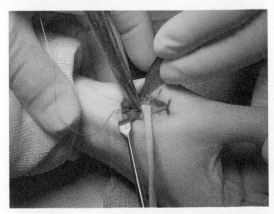

Fig. 16. Final suturing of tensioned graft back to FCR.

Table 2
Preliminary data for CMC arthroplasty with GraftJacket study

		FCR	GraftJacket
Recovery time (d)	n	30	26
	Avg	21.83	18.34
Grip strength (N)	n	17	14
	Avg	37.41	46.41
Pinch strength (N)	n	16	12
	Avg	8.88	10.33
Three-finger pinch strength (N)	n	9	9
	Avg	8.22	8.66
Tip pinch strength (N)	n	4	2
	Avg	6.5	7.5

Abbreviations: Avg, average; N, Newtons.

The authors' series consisted of 79 patients who underwent CMC arthroplasty with the split-FCR LRTI method versus trapeziectomy with GraftJacket suspensionplasty. At the time of chart review, 56 of the patients were eligible for inclusion in the study with 13 patients lost to inadequate follow-up. The parameters were analyzed within 1 year of surgery to compare the two techniques. In all patients, the amount of time, in weeks, to full recovery from the surgery was reviewed. Full recovery was defined as time until returned to work (in days), or, in those patients who were retired or did not work, time returned to normal daily activities, as reported by patients at follow-up. The other endpoints for the study included grip strength, three-finger pinch strength, and tip-pinch strength.

Preliminary data for each of the parameters are shown in **Table 2**. No statistical difference was identified between either study arm for every category. No major complications were noted in either group, except there were two cases of transient radial sensory neuritis in each group. In short, the preliminary data provide further evidence that GraftJacket acellular dermal allograft interposition for CMC arthroplasty is a safe and effective alternative to FCR interposition.

SUMMARY

The three core principles for surgery for CMC arthritis include (1) removal of diseased joint surfaces, (2) reconstruction of ligamentous stabilizers, and (3) preservation of the arthroplasty space. Of the myriad surgical solutions investigated for the treatment of CMC arthritis of the thumb, the ligament reconstruction interposition arthroplasty has proved durable at long-term follow-up. The many variations and adaptations

of this technique, reviewed in this article, illustrate that it is an evolving procedure. The use of ligament reconstruction and suspensionplasty with acellular dermal allograft tendon forgoes the potential morbidity of autologous tendon harvest and satisfies the three core principles for surgery for CMC arthritis. The authors submit that it is a safe and effective alternative to traditional ligament reconstruction interposition arthroplasty.

REFERENCES

1. Eaton RG, Littler JW. Ligament reconstruction for the painful thumb carpometacarpal joint. J Bone Joint Surg 1973;55:1655–66.
2. Chaisson CE, Zhang Y, McAlindon TE, et al. Radiographic hand osteoarthritis: incidence, patterns, and influence of pre-existing disease in a population based sample. J Rheumatol 1997;24(7):1337–43.
3. Swigart C, Eaton R, Gllickel S, et al. Splinting in the treatment of arthritis of the first carpometacarpal joint. J Hand Surg Am 1999;24:86–91.
4. Armstrong AL, Hunter JB, Davis TR. The prevalence of degenerative arthritis of the base of the thumb in post-menopausal women. J Hand Surg Br 1994; 19(3):340–1.
5. Sodha S, Ring D, Zurakowski D, et al. Prevalence of osteoarthrosis of the trapeziometacarpal joint. J Bone Joint Surg Am 2005;87(12):2614–8.
6. Matullo KS, Ilyas A, Thoder JJ. CMC arthroplasty of the thumb: a review. Hand (N Y) 2007;2(4):232–9.
7. Eaton RG, Glickel SZ. Trapeziometacarpal osteoarthritis. Staging as a rationale for treatment. Hand Clin 1987;3(4):455–71.
8. Bettinger PC, Linscheid RL, Berger RA, et al. An anatomic study of the stabilizing ligaments of the trapezium and trapeziometacarpal joint. J Hand Surg Am 1999;24(4):786–98.
9. Tomaino M, King J, Leit M. Thumb basal joint arthritis. In: Green DP, Hotchkiss RN, Penderson WC, et al, editors. Green's operative hand surgery. 5th edition. Amsterdam: Elsevier; 2007. p. 461–86.
10. Burton RI, Pellegrini VD Jr. Surgical management of basal joint arthritis of the thumb. Part II. Ligament reconstruction with tendon interposition arthroplasty. J Hand Surg Am 1986;11(3):324–32.
11. Tomaino MM, Pellegrini VD, Burton RI. Arthroplasty of the basaljoint of the thumb. Long-term follow-up after ligament reconstruction with tendon interposition. J Bone Joint Surg Am 1995;77:346–55.
12. Gervis WH. Excision of the trapezium for osteoarthritis of the trapezio-metacarpal joint. J Bone Joint Surg Br 1949;31(4):537–9.
13. Gervis WH, Wells T. A review of excision of the trapezium for osteoarthritis of the trapezio-metacarpal

joint after twenty-five years. J Bone Joint Surg Br 1973;55(1):56–7.

14. Kuhns CA, Emerson ET, Meals RA. Hematoma and distraction arthroplasty for thumb basal joint osteoarthritis: a prospective, single-surgeon study including outcomes measures. J Hand Surg Am 2003;28(3):381–9.

15. Eaton RG, Glickel SZ, Littler JW. Tendon interposition arthroplasty for degenerative arthritis of the trapeziometacarpal joint of the thumb. J Hand Surg Am 1985;10:645–54.

16. Froimson AI. Tendon arthroplasty of the trapeziometacarpal joint. Clin Orthop Relat Res 1970;70:191–9.

17. Menon J, Schoene HR, Hohl JC. Trapeziometacarpal arthritis-results of tendon interpositional arthroplasty. J Hand Surg Am 1981;6(5):442–6.

18. Kriegs-Au G, Petje G, Fojtl E, et al. Ligament reconstruction with or without tendon interposition to treat primary thumb carpometacarpal osteoarthritis. J Bone Joint Surg 2005;87:78–85.

19. Soejima O, Hanamura T, Kikuta T, et al. Suspension-plasty with the abductor pollicis longus tendon for osteoarthritis in the carpometacarpal joint of the thumb. J Hand Surg Am 2006;31(3):425–8.

20. Gerwin M, Griffith A, Weiland AJ, et al. Ligament reconstruction basal joint arthroplasty without tendon interposition. Clin Orthop Relat Res 1997; 342:42–5.

21. Diao E. Trapezio-metacarpal arthritis. Trapezium excision and ligament reconstruction not including the LRTI arthroplasty. Hand Clin 2001;17(2):223–36, ix.

22. Naidu SH, Poole J, Horne A. Entire flexor carpi radialis tendon harvest for thumb carpometacarpal arthroplasty alters wrist kinetics. J Hand Surg Am 2006;31:1171–5.

23. de la Caffiniere JY, Aucouturier P. Trapezio-metacarpal arthroplasty by total prosthesis. Hand 1979; 11(1):41–6.

24. Badia A, Sambandam SN. Total joint arthroplasty in the treatment of advanced stages of thumb carpometacarpal joint osteoarthritis. J Hand Surg Am 2006;32(10):1605 e1–e13.

25. de la Caffinière JY. [Long-term results of the total trapezio-metacarpal prosthesis in osteoarthritis of the thumb]. Rev Chir Orthop Reparatrice Appar Mot 1991;77(5):312–21 [in French].

26. Lemoine S, Wavreille G, Alnot JY, et al. groupe GUEPAR. Second generation GUEPAR total arthroplasty of the thumb basal joint: 50 months follow-up in 84 cases. Orthop Traumatol Surg Res 2009;95(1):63–9.

27. Pellegrini VD Jr, Burton RI. Surgical management of basal joint arthritis of the thumb. Part I. Long-term results of silicone implant arthroplasty. J Hand Surg Am 1986;11(3):309–24.

28. Eaton RG. Replacement of the trapezium for arthritis of the basal articulations: a new technique with stabilization by tenodesis. J Bone Joint Surg Am 1979;61:76–82.

29. Creighton JJ Jr, Steichen JB, Strickland JW. Long-term evaluation of Silastic trapezial arthroplasty in patients with osteoarthritis. J Hand Surg Am 1991; 16(3):510–9.

30. Greenberg JA, Mosher JF Jr, Fatti JF. X-ray changes after expanded polytetrafluoroethylene (Gore-Tex) interpositional arthroplasty. J Hand Surg Am 1997; 22(4):658–63.

31. Muermans S, Coenen L. Interpositional arthroplasty with Gore-Tex, Marlex or tendon for osteoarthritis of the trapeziometacarpal joint. A retrospective comparative study. J Hand Surg Br 1998;23(1):64–8.

32. Belcher HJ, Zic R. Adverse effect of porcine collagen interposition after trapeziectomy: a comparative study. J Hand Surg Br 2001;26(2):159–64.

33. Beniker D, McQuillan D, Livesey S, et al. The use of acellular dermal matrix as a scaffold for periosteum replacement. Orthopedics 2003;26(Suppl 5): s591–6.

34. Lee DK. Achilles tendon repair with acellular tissue graft augmentation in neglected ruptures. J Foot Ankle Surg 2007;46(6):451–5.

35. Lee MS. GraftJacket augmentation of chronic Achilles tendon ruptures. Orthopedics 2004; 27(1 Suppl):s151–3.

36. Bond JL, Dopirak RM, Higgins J, et al. Arthroscopic replacement of massive, irreparable rotator cuff tears using a GraftJacket allograft: technique and preliminary results. Arthroscopy 2008;24(4):403–9 e1.

37. Adams JE, Merten SM, Steinmann SP. Arthroscopic interposition arthroplasty of the first carpometacarpal joint. J Hand Surg Eur Vol 2007;32(3):268–74.

38. Bhatia DN, van Rooyen KS, du Toit DF, et al. Arthroscopic technique of interposition arthroplasty of the glenohumeral joint. Arthroscopy 2006;22(5):570 e1–e5.

39. Adams JE, Zobitz ME, Reach JS Jr, et al. Rotator cuff repair using an acellular dermal matrix graft: an in vivo study in a canine model. Arthroscopy 2006; 22(7):700–9.

40. Kokkalis ZT, Zanaros G, Sotereanos DG. Ligament reconstruction with tendon interposition using an acellular dermal allograft for thumb carpometacarpal arthritis. Tech Hand Up Extrem Surg 2009;13: 41–6.

41. Kokkalis ZT, Zanaros G, Weiser RW, et al. Trapezium resection with suspension and interposition arthroplasty using acellular dermal allograft for thumb carpometacarpal arthritis. J Hand Surg Am 2009;34(6): 1029–36.

Headless Compression Screw Fixation of Scaphoid Fractures

John R. Fowler, MD[a], Asif M. Ilyas, MD[b,c],*

KEYWORDS

- Scaphoid fracture • Headless screw • Herbert screw
- Acutrak screw • Twinfix screw

The scaphoid is the most commonly fractured carpal bone and most common hand fracture, accounting for 60% and 11% of fractures respectively.[1] The annual incidence of scaphoid fractures is estimated to be 38 to 43 per 100,000[2,3]; patients are an average age of 25.[4,5] Of these fractures, 70% to 80% occur at the scaphoid waist and 10% to 20% involve the proximal third.[6] Inadequately treated scaphoid fractures are prone to develop into malunions and nonunions that can cause pain, altered carpal kinematics, diminished range of motion, disuse osteopenia, and decreased grip strength, and result in dorsal intercalary segmental instability and degenerative changes.[1]

Nondisplaced and minimally displaced fractures of the scaphoid can be treated successfully with cast immobilization. The prolonged immobilization required for nonoperative treatment of scaphoid fractures can pose significant morbidity as well as a socioeconomic burden to the patient.[2] Scaphoid fractures are a significant problem in college and professional athletics, with the incidence of scaphoid fractures in college football players estimated to be 1 in 100.[7] Young, active patients, or those who cannot entertain prolonged absence from their occupations may prefer definitive operative fixation to prevent prolonged immobilization and to facilitate return to work or sports.[4]

APPLIED ANATOMY OF THE SCAPHOID

Scaphoid is derived from the Greek work *scaphe*, for skiff or boat,[1,8] although some think it more resembles a twisted peanut.[9] The scaphoid has a palmar concave and ulnar concave curvature.[8] The proximal, distal, medial, and half of the lateral surface are covered with cartilage.[1] The blood supply to the scaphoid has been extensively studied. The distal pole is richly vascularized by direct branches from the radial artery.[8] Most of the intraosseous blood supply arises from the perforating branches of the radial artery that enter dorsally on the dorsal ridge and dorsal tubercle.[1] These vessels enter the scaphoid at a nonarticular portion, through a foramina on the dorsal ridge at the level of the scaphoid waist.[10] Retrograde flow allows dorsal branches to supply the proximal pole.[1] Consequently, fractures involving the proximal pole are at risk for osteonecrosis and nonunion.[11] The distal pole also receives blood supply from the superficial palmar branch of the radial artery.[1,10]

The scaphoid has numerous ligamentous attachments, leading to the characteristic humpback deformity when fracture occurs.[11] The scapholunate interosseous ligament attaches along the ulnar aspect of the proximal pole. The proximal pole, therefore, extends because of its attachment to the lunate while the distal fragment remains

a Temple University Hospital, 3401 North Broad Street, Philadelphia, PA, USA
b Rothman Institute–Hand & Wrist Service, 925 Chestnut Street, Philadelphia, PA 19107, USA
c Orthopaedic Surgery, Thomas Jefferson University Hospital, Philadelphia, PA, USA
* Corresponding author. Rothman Institute–Hand & Wrist Service, 925 Chestnut Street, Philadelphia, PA 19107.
E-mail address: aimd2001@yahoo.com

Hand Clin 26 (2010) 351–361
doi:10.1016/j.hcl.2010.04.005

flexed because of its attachment to the trapezium and trapezoid via the scaphotrapezial ligament.[1,11] Just proximal to the attachment of the scaphotrapezial ligament is the attachment of the dorsal intercarpal ligament along the dorsum of the scaphoid.[1] The scaphocapitate ligament is directly palmar to the distal pole of the scaphoid.[1] The long radiolunate ligament passes along the palmar aspect of the proximal part of the scaphoid as it inserts on the lunate.[1] The radioscaphocapitate ligament inserts on the waist of the scaphoid.[1]

The anatomy of the scaphoid contributes greatly to the risk of malunion and nonunion. Scaphoid fractures unite by primary bone healing without external callus. The scaphoid is almost completely covered with articular cartilage, limiting the amount of surface area for bone contact and healing. Owing to its intra-articular location, synovial fluid may pass between the fracture fragments, delaying healing.[4,7]

TREATMENT CONSIDERATIONS

The reported rates of nonunion for scaphoid fractures range from 5% to 25%, with displaced fractures carrying a higher risk.[1] Displacement of more than 1 mm, fracture of the proximal pole, history of osteonecrosis, vertical oblique fracture pattern, and nicotine use are all risk factors for nonunion.[1] Malunion and nonunions present difficult management problems. They can result in pain, altered carpal kinematics, diminished range of motion, disuse osteopenia, and decreased grip strength and result in dorsal intercalary segmental instability and degenerative changes.[1,7,10,11] Most investigators have recommended internal fixation of all displaced scaphoid fractures and several also recommend internal fixation of nondisplaced fractures in young, active individuals who require full use of their hands for work or sports.[2,5,7,11] Prolonged inability to return to work or sports can compromise a worker's employment or an athlete's scholarship.[7] Additionally, patients treated nonoperatively with cast immobilization require frequent office visits and radiographic evaluations to monitor for evidence of fracture union and avoid malunion or nonunion.[2] Patient dissatisfaction secondary to prolonged immobilization, frequent clinic visits, and radiographic monitoring is common.[7]

Approximately 95% of acute nondisplaced scaphoid fractures will eventually achieve successful union with cast immobilization.[12] The average time to union varies greatly, depending on the location of the fracture. Distal one-third fractures demonstrate radiographic union in an average of 6 to 8 weeks, middle one-third fractures demonstrate healing in 8 to 12 weeks, and some proximal pole fractures can require 12 to 23 weeks of immobilization to achieve union.[13] Cooney[14] reviewed 45 acute scaphoid fractures at the Mayo Clinic from 1976 to 1978[15] and found that 30 (94%) of 32 nondisplaced fractures achieved radiographic union whereas only 7 (54%) of 13 displaced fractures achieved union.

The major advantages of internal fixation of scaphoid fractures include limited immobilization and the potential for earlier to return to sports and work.[11] Capo and colleagues[16] noted that cast immobilization does not eliminate micromotion at the fracture site and does not alter the biologic environment to promote healing. Rigid internal fixation may allow early mobilization, decreased time to union, and improved range of motion, and can lead to a more rapid functional recovery.[17] Bond and colleagues,[18] in a prospective analysis, randomized 25 military recruits with acute nondisplaced fractures of the scaphoid waist to either cast immobilization or percutaneous cannulated Acutrak (Acumed, Beaverton, OR, USA) screw fixation. The patients in the screw fixation group achieved a faster time to union (7 weeks vs 12 weeks) and a faster return to work (8 weeks vs 15 weeks). There was no significant difference between the 2 groups in regard to range of motion or grip strength.

McQueen and colleagues,[5] in a recent prospective randomized trial, randomly allocated 60 consecutive patients with scaphoid waist fractures to percutaneous fixation with a cannulated Acutrak screw (Acumed) or cast immobilization. Patients who underwent percutaneous fixation showed a faster time to union (9.2 weeks vs 13.9 weeks, $P<.001$). There was a trend toward a higher rate of nonunion in the nonoperative group (4 of 30 vs 1 of 30), although this was not statistically significant. Patients treated with percutaneous internal fixation had a more rapid return of function and return to sports and work compared with those managed nonoperatively with a low complication rate. The authors recommended that all active patients should be offered percutaneous stabilization for fractures of the waist of the scaphoid.

Similarly, the goals of percutaneous fixation of stable scaphoid fractures include early motion and return to activity while improving union rates, avoiding problems associated with prolonged immobilization, and minimizing morbidity from surgical dissection. Percutaneous screw fixation is primarily indicated for minimally or nondisplaced scaphoid waist and proximal pole fractures. Displacement of more than 1 mm is an indication for open reduction to obtain anatomic alignment.[19]

TREATMENT OPTIONS

Cast immobilization has been the mainstay of treatment for more than 100 years. As previously mentioned, nondisplaced fractures have a high rate of union when treated with cast immobilization. The position of the wrist in the cast, inclusion of the elbow in the cast, and inclusion of the thumb in the cast (thumb spica) are all points of controversy and have recently been shown to not significantly affect the rates of union.[1] Before the introduction of the headless compression screw by Herbert, fractures requiring operative intervention were reduced under open technique and stabilized using Kirschner wires (K-wires) or AO lag screws.

Cosio and Camp[20] reported on fixation of scaphoid nonunion with K-wires and documented a union rate of 77%. Percutaneous internal fixation of scaphoid fractures using a headed cannulated screw was first performed in 1962 by Streli.[4] Wozasek and Moser[21] published a series of more than 200 patients treated with the headed cannulated screw, with a union rate of 89% for acute fractures and 82% in nonunions. Sclerotic nonunions, however, united in only 43% of cases. Ledoux and colleagues[22] used Herbert screws and a retrograde volar approach to achieve 100% union in 23 cases with, on average, only 15 days of immobilization.

The headless compression screw, developed by Herbert,[23] decreased the incidence of arthrosis owing to prominence of the screw head. Whipple[24] modified the Herbert screw by developing a cannulated version to allow for more accurate percutaneous screw placement and arthroscopy-assisted reduction. The use of a headless cannulated screw with placement of a percutaneous guidewire from the volar approach was popularized by several investigators during the 1990s.[4]

A major limitation of the first generation headless compression screws was the need for significant exposure to apply the scaphoid clamps and targeting jigs necessary for their insertion. The concern over soft tissue stripping and vascular compromise encouraged the development of newer screws and percutaneous techniques in use today.[25] The use of a headless variable pitch screw for percutaneous fixation was first reported by Ledoux and colleagues[22] in 1995 and Inoue and colleagues[13] in 1997, with both investigators reporting excellent results. These promising results, combined with improvements in fluoroscopy and implants, has led many surgeons to use percutaneous fixation with second generation headless compression screws as the procedure of choice for operative treatment of scaphoid fractures. Another advancement in the operative treatment of scaphoid fractures was the use of arthroscopy to assist and confirm reduction of the fracture and ensure extra-articular placement of the screws.[26]

SCAPHOID SCREWS
First Generation

The Herbert Screw[23] was the original, noncannulated, headless compression screw with a second set of threads in place of the screw head. The design allowed for a reduction in the overall diameter of the implant, fixation of both fragments, and avoidance of metal on the articular surface. To apply compression, the thread on the leading edge of the screw has a greater pitch than at the trailing end, leading to compression. The impetus for such a screw design was the observation that the main factor related to failure of scaphoid fracture union was the lack of a suitable implant that would permit compression and fixation in cancellous bone. The use of K-wires did not produce rigid fixation, often led to distraction, required continued immobilization, and necessitated a second operation for hardware removal.[23] Because the standard cancellous or lag screws led to a significant number of failures, Herbert believed the ideal implant was an intramedullary device using a compression jig that could provide fixation and compression across the fracture.[23] The Herbert screw was designed to apply compression through the differential in pitch between the proximal and distal threads of the screw. By today's standards, Herbert used an extensile approach, fully exposing the scaphoid along its volar surface by retracting the flexor carpi radialis tendon and incising the capsule. The distal pole of the scaphoid was also exposed, followed by application of a targeting jig to apply compression across the fracture site. The fracture site was debrided and iliac crest bone graft was applied, if necessary (performed in only 2 acute fractures, but in all nonunions).

Herbert performed internal fixation via a volar approach centered on the scaphoid tubercle in 158 patients with either acute scaphoid fractures or nonunions from 1977–1981 and achieved a 100% radiographic union rate in the acute fractures (43 fractures) and 83% in the nonunions (115 fractures).[23] The average age in this series was 24.8, 94% of the patients were male, and the dominant hand was affected in 59%. Postoperative immobilization was instituted in 15 of 43 acute fractures that the investigators felt had associated ligamentous injury and in 28 of 115 nonunions. The average time to return to work was 5.5 weeks for patients not involved in worker's compensation and 6.8 weeks in patients with worker's compensation. Herbert identified several risk factors for nonunion in this series, including time to treatment (many of the nonunions were treated more than 18 months after the injury) and proximal pole fractures with sclerotic bone.

Biomechanical studies and a retrospective series by Trumble and colleagues[27] have shown that placement of the screw in the central one-third of the scaphoid significantly reduced time to union when compared with screws placed in the outer thirds. Accurate placement of the non-cannulated Herbert screw, however, is difficult despite the use of a jig. Screws inserted from an unfavorable position are often difficult to reorient. The use of a jig also requires the division of the entire volar capsule to place the device onto the proximal pole of the scaphoid, potentially damaging the vascular supply to the scaphoid.[28] In response to these challenges, the Herbert-Whipple screw, a cannulated Herbert screw (**Fig. 1**), was developed to address the aforementioned concerns of the Herbert screw. The screw diameter was increased to 2.5 mm to allow cannulation and insertion over a guidewire.[29] The leading threads are self-tapping to ease insertion and the pitch differential between the leading and trailing threads was designed to generate interfragmentary compression. Additionally, "pre"-compression can be obtained if the optional guide jig or a tong is used.[30]

Second Generation

Building on the success of the first generation of headless compression screws, a new generation has evolved, building on the principles of strong cannulated compression of cancellous bones but focusing on increased compressive strength and versatility.

The Acutrak screw (Acumed) is a headless, highly polished, tapered, self-tapping, fully threaded, cannulated device designed to provide interfragmentary compression (**Fig. 2**). The variable pitch across the entire screw causes gradual compression during insertion and avoids the lag-screw requirement of smooth shank at the fracture site. The screws are titanium and available in mini and standard sizes. The mini screws are available in lengths from 10.0 to 26.0 mm in 2.0-mm increments. The standard size screws are available in lengths from 12.5 to 30.0 mm in 2.5-mm increments. Standard screws have a distal tip diameter of 3.3 mm that progress to 3.8 to 4.6 mm depending on the length of screw chosen. The mini-size screw has a distal tip diameter of 2.8 mm and progresses to 3.2 to 3.6 mm depending on screw length. Because it is completely threaded, there is a greater surface area for fixation between the bone and the screw. Its conical shape also may be an advantage with regard to avoiding pistoning within the scaphoid.[31]

The 3.0-mm and 2.4-mm Headless Compression Screws (Synthes, Paoli, PA, USA) are self-drilling, cannulated, and self-tapping headless screws available in titanium or stainless steel at screw lengths of 9 to 40 mm (**Fig. 3**). A 1.1-mm threaded or nonthreaded guidewire is also used. The distal threads are either long (40% of screw length) or short (20% of screw length) depending on the location of the fracture. The screwdriver

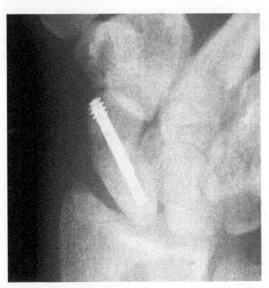

Fig. 1. Herbert-Whipple screw.

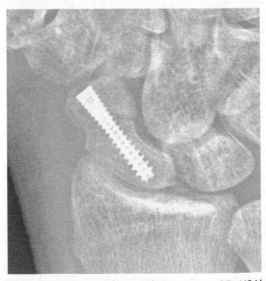

Fig. 2. Acutrak screw (Acumed, Beaverton, OR, USA).

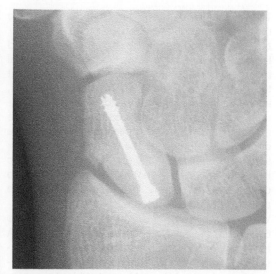

Fig. 3. A 3.0 AO Headless compression screw (Synthes, Paoli, PA, USA).

has a star-drive and compression sleeve. When the tip of the compression sleeve contacts the bone the fracture gap is compressed as though it were a headed lag screw. The design allows for surgeon-controlled compression. Following compression of the fracture, the compression sleeve is held stationary while the screwdriver is turned, thus counter-sinking the screw head and holding the compression.

The Stryker TwinFix (Stryker, Kalamazoo MI, USA) is a self-tapping, cannulated, headless compression screw (**Fig. 4**). It has a shaft diameter

of 3.2 mm, screw lengths of 14 to 34 mm, and allows placement of a 1-mm threaded K-wire. The distal thread has a diameter of 3.35 mm and the proximal thread has a diameter of 4.07 mm. Independent rotation of the distal threads allows for additional dynamic adjustable interfragmentary compression once the screw has been fully inserted. The screwdriver is locked when inserting the screw, causing the screw head and screw foot to turn simultaneously. When the reamer below the head reaches the cortex, precompression of the fracture occurs. When the screw head is completely submerged in bone, the screwdriver is unlocked, allowing only the screw foot (distal threads) to turn. A quarter turn of the screwdriver further compresses the fracture.

The Integra Kompressor (Integra, Plainsboro, NJ, USA) is a titanium self-tapping, cannulated, headless, 2-piece compression screw (**Fig. 5**). It is offered in two sizes: Standard and Mini. The Standard screws are available from 14 to 34 mm and have a 4.0 mm leading diameter and a 5.0 mm trailing diameter. The Mini screws are available from 10 to 26 mm and have a 2.8 mm leading diameter and a 3.6 mm trailing diameter. The Kompressor screws arrive in two parts and are are assembled on the backtable with an insertion jig into a single unit. The system allows placement of the screw over a guidewire into the desired

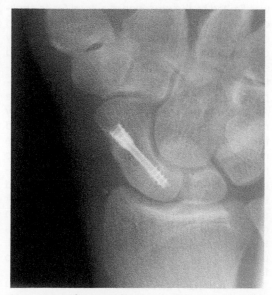

Fig. 4. A Twinfix screw (Stryker, Kalamazoo, MI, USA).

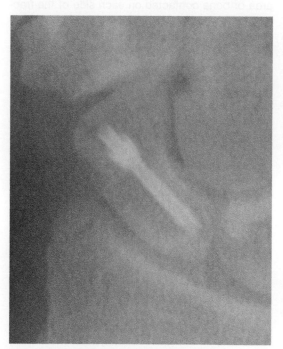

Fig. 5. A Kompressor screw (Integra, Plainsboro, NJ, USA).

position followed by manually applied compression. The outer driver on the assembled jig rotates the trailing head over the fixed leading end resulting in additional compression across the fracture site.

BIOMECHANICAL STUDIES

Second generation scaphoid compression screws have been designed to ensure accurate placement within the bone, maximize compression forces across the fracture site, and increase the number of loads to failure. Biomechanical studies have shown that wider screws better resist lateral displacement, which is proportional to the radius of the screw to the fourth power.[1] Trumble and colleagues[28] and McCallister and colleagues[32] demonstrated that screws should be placed centrally within the middle third of the proximal pole of the scaphoid on both the anteroposterior and lateral views. Dodds and colleagues[33] found that long screws placed down the central axis of the scaphoid, deep into subchondral bone, provided optimal fixation. The most stable configuration was a long screw augmented with parallel K-wire, but this configuration was not significantly stronger than a long screw alone. Gutow[4] explained that although the rigidity of the fixation of a metal screw is directly proportional to the radius to the fourth power, the rigidity of the bone-screw construct is directly proportional to the surface area of bone contacted on each side of the fracture by the screw. The surface area of cancellous bone resisting bending is a function of the diameter of the screw and the length of the screw on each side of the fracture. Although the longest possible screw length may impart optimal biomechanical stability, scaphoid screws should be no longer than 4 mm less than the measured scaphoid length (leaving at least 2 mm of bone coverage at both ends of the scaphoid). Screw prominence at the articular surface will lead to unacceptable hardware irritation and subsequent chondral wear.

Several authors have compared the biomechanical properties of the first generation Herbert screws and Herbert-Whipple screws to the second generation headless compression screws.[30–38] In general, the results have favored the second generation screws in both the compression force across the fracture site and the load/cycles to failure of the screws. Toby and colleagues,[31] using cadaveric scaphoid bone, found that the Herbert-Whipple screw and the Acutrak screw required nearly twice as many loading cycles to create fracture fragment displacement than the standard Herbert screw.

The investigators also demonstrated that the mode of failure differed between the first generation and second generation screws. Herbert and Herbert-Whipple screws failed at the proximal threads whereas cannulated AO screws failed at the distal thread insertion. The Acutrak screws, interestingly, demonstrated no catastrophic failures, but instead gradually loosened. In a sawbone model, Hausman and colleagues[30] found the compressive forces of the Acutrak and Twinfix screws to be significantly greater than the classic Herbert screw, Herber-Whipple screw, and the cannulated AO screw. The authors found the average compressive forces of the AO, Herbert-Whipple, Acutrak, and TwinFix screws to be 6.8 N, 2.0 N, 7.6 N, and 8.0 N, respectively. A time plot of the compression forces over a 30-second period also found a decay in the compression force for the AO and Herbert-Whipple screws, but less so for the Acutrak and TwinFix screws. Lo and colleagues[34] echoed those findings, demonstrating that classic Herbert screws lose most of their compressive forces over time and more specifically after the targeting guide was removed, retaining only 38% of the peak compression achieved during insertion.

Adla and colleagues[35] compared the Mini-Acutrak, Herbert-Whipple, and AO 2.0-mm and 3.0-mm cancellous screws in a foam model. The authors found no significant difference in the compression forces generated by the Mini-Acutrak and Herbert-Whipple screws. The Mini-Acutrak and Herbert-Whipple screws did generate significantly more compression force than the 2.0-mm AO screw. The 3.0-mm AO cancellous screw had the highest compression forces, but it was limited by the presence of a head for its application in scaphoid fixation. Beadel and colleagues[36] found that the interfragmentary compression generated by the Acutrak Standard screw was significantly greater and more consistent than that generated by either a Herbert-Whipple screw or Acutrak Mini (Acumed) screws. The Acutrak Standard screw produced significantly more compression across a simulated scaphoid fracture (152 N) than either the Herbert-Whipple (103 N) or Acutrak Mini screws (92 N) and it was more consistent, as reflected by the lower standard deviation. Wheeler and McLoughlin[37] noted superior mechanical characteristics of the Acutrak screw when compared with first generation compression screws in every mode the authors tested, including compression force generated, pullout strength, load to failure, and torque to failure.

Although many investigators have found differences in the compression forces generated by different screws, Newport and colleagues[38] found no significant difference when comparing the Herbert-Whipple screw, Howmedica (Howmedica Orthopedics, Rutherford, NJ, USA) Universal Compression Screw, AO 2.7-mm and 3.0-mm screws, and classic Herbert screw. It should be noted that although most investigators have found a statistical difference between the compressive forces generated and maintained by first and second generation scaphoid screws, the clinical significance of a 1-Newton difference in compressive force remains to be determined.

SURGICAL TECHNIQUE
Volar Open

The classic Russe approach is an open volar approach that yields excellent visualization with less risk of damage to the blood supply, which primarily enters dorsally.[1] The volar Russe approach allows inspection of the entire volar surface of the scaphoid, but can lead to scarring, decreased wrist extension, potential damage to the radiocarpal ligaments, and inability to assess the dorsal scapholunate ligament.[1] Herbert believed it was the best approach for distal two-thirds fractures that are not amenable to closed reduction or percutaneous techniques.[39] Similarly, it is the authors' preferred technique for "hump-back" scaphoid malunion or nonunion correction, assuming there is no osteonecrosis present.

The patient is placed supine on the operating table with the arm abducted onto a radiolucent arm board. A rolled towel is placed under the supinated wrist to allow for adequate wrist extension. A longitudinal incision is made just radial to the flexor carpi ulnaris, which is then retracted to the ulnar side. The incision is carried distally over the wrist crease and scaphoid tubercle of the scaphoid in an oblique radially angled fashion. The volar capsule is incised in longitudinal fashion, taking care not to damage the radioscaphocapitate ligament. The nonarticular portion of the proximal trapezium can be resected to gain access to the distal scaphoid, if needed. The fracture is reduced, bone grafted if necessary, and pinned with guidewires and/or additional K-wires.

Dorsal Open

The dorsal approach is the preferred approach for proximal pole fractures.[1] It is a straightforward technique that allows excellent visualization of the proximal pole of the scaphoid, permits visualization of a reliable starting point for screw placement within the central axis of the scaphoid, allows examination of the scapholunate ligament,

and avoids potential damage to the volar radiocarpal ligaments and scaphotrapezial articulation.[17]

A longitudinal incision is placed just distal and ulnar to Lister's tubercle. The extensor retinaculum is incised in a longitudinal fashion to allow retraction of the extensor pollicis longus tendon exiting the third dorsal compartments and development of the interval between the third and fourth dorsal compartments. The wrist capsule is incised longitudinally, with care taken not to injure the scapholunate ligament deep to the capsule. Excessive dissection distally should be resisted to avoid disturbance of the dorsal blood supply that inserts at the distal dorsal ridge. The proximal pole of the scaphoid will be readily visualized by volar-flexing the wrist.

Percutaneous

Percutaneous fixation is becoming a more popular alternative to prolonged immobilization for nondisplaced fractures (Fig. 6A).[1] In a study by Bond and Shin,[40] patients treated with percutaneous fixation were able to return to work at an average of 8 weeks, compared with 15 weeks in the cast group. This method is reserved for fractures that are nondisplaced or those that can be anatomically reduced using closed or arthroscopic means.[1]

For the volar percutaneous approach, the distal aspect of the scaphoid is used for the entry point. Once satisfactory reduction of the fracture has been achieved, the tubercle of the scaphoid, which becomes more prominent in full radial deviation of the wrist, is palpated and marked on the skin. A short incision (3–5 mm) is made over the scaphotrapezial joint, and the distal pole of the scaphoid is exposed. The guidewire is started volar at the tubercle and aimed dorsally, aiming the guide toward the proximal pole of the scaphoid (approximately 45 degrees dorsally and 45 degrees ulnarly, with the wrist in neutral), the guidewire is inserted slowly under fluoroscopy (see Fig. 6B). Overhanging trapezium is sometimes removed to achieve a good starting point. The volar approach does not violate the proximal cartilaginous surface of the scaphoid.

With the dorsal percutaneous approach, the proximal pole of the scaphoid is used as the entry point. The wrist is placed in maximum flexion and slight ulnar deviation to maximize ease of entry of the guidewire into the proximal pole. By pronating, flexing, and ulnarly deviating the wrist, the scaphoid can be viewed with fluoroscopy as a cylinder. A guidewire that is introduced down the center of this cylinder will be placed along the central anatomic axis of the scaphoid. The wire is advanced across the scaphoid fracture site. Before

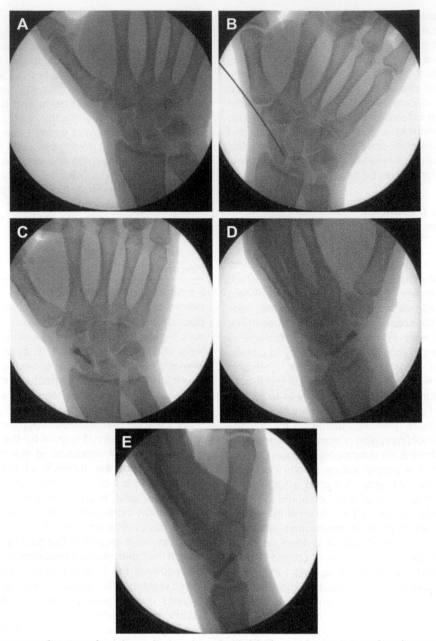

Fig. 6. Percutaneous fixation of a (A) nondisplaced scaphoid. (B) The guidewire is introduced approximately 45 dorsally and 45 ulnarly. After measuring the guidewire, overdrilling, the screw is placed. Final radiographs including a (C) scaphoid view, (D) oblique view, and (E) lateral views should be taken to confirm fracture reduction and appropriate screw position.

reaming, a second guidewire can be placed parallel to the first guidewire for antirotation control.[19]

The guidewire is measured and then overdrilled with a cannulated drill bit. The screw should be placed so as to be at least 2 mm below the articular surface on both ends. Final radiographs should be taken to confirm appropriate fracture reduction and central screw position on

a Scaphoid view, oblique view, and lateral view (see **Fig. 6**C, D, and E).

Outcomes

In general, internal fixation of scaphoid fractures has led to at least equivalent rates of union to cast immobilization in nondisplaced fractures and higher rates of union in displaced fractures. In addition, internal fixation may result in more rapid union of fractures and faster return to work and activities. Most outcome data for the second generation headless scaphoid compression screws is based on use of the Acutrak screw.

Nondisplaced

Adolfsson and colleagues[41] randomized 25 patients with nondisplaced scaphoid fractures to percutaneous fixation with Acutrak screw and 28 patients to below-elbow cast immobilization for 10 weeks. There was no difference between the groups in regard to rate of union or time to union. Patients who underwent internal fixation had a significantly better range of motion postoperatively, but there were no differences in grip strength. The investigators felt that internal fixation showed no adverse effects on healing. Bond and colleagues[18] studied a military population with nondisplaced scaphoid fractures. Eleven patients received percutaneous cannulated screw fixation with an Acutrak screw and 14 received cast immobilization. The average time to fracture union in the screw fixation group was 7 weeks compared with 12 weeks in the cast immobilization group ($P = .0003$). The average time until the patients returned to work was 8 weeks compared with 15 weeks in the cast immobilization group ($P = .0001$). There was no significant difference in the range of motion of the wrist or in grip strength at the 2-year follow-up evaluation. Overall patient satisfaction was high in both groups.

Haddad and Goddard[42] used Acutrak screws to treat 15 patients with non- or minimally displaced acute scaphoid fractures with immediate postoperative mobilization. A subjective functional assessment at 3 months gave an excellent result in 13 patients and a good result in 2. Return to work ranged from 4 to 37 days depending on the patients' occupation and return to active sports from 43 to 75 days. Full flexion, extension, and ulnar deviation were achieved in all patients at 6 weeks, and radial deviation was equal to the contralateral side after 3 months in 12 patients, and after 4 months in another 2. Bedi and colleagues[17] reviewed 18 patients with nondisplaced scaphoid fractures treated with percutaneous internal fixation using Acutrak screws, achieving union in 17 (94%) of 18 patients. No significant difference was noted in grip strength, flexion, or ulnar deviation between the injured and noninjured wrist, but patients did lose an average of 6 degrees of wrist extension on the operative side.

Displaced

Chen and colleagues[43] reviewed 11 patients with acute displaced scaphoid fractures who underwent percutaneous internal fixation via a volar approach: 100% achieved radiographic union in a mean of 10.6 weeks with 100% good or excellent results and 100% returning to work by 12 weeks. The results from this series are in stark contrast to the results obtained in Cooney's series[15] of displaced scaphoid fractures, which achieved a union rate of 54% when treated with cast immobilization. Rettig and colleagues[44] reviewed 14 acute displaced scaphoid fractures treated with K-wires and Herbert screws. Thirteen of 14 achieved radiographic union at an average of 11.5 weeks. The 1 nonunion occurred in a patient treated with 2 K-wires. The investigators found no statistical difference between the K-wire and Herbert screw groups.

Herbert screws

Jeon and colleagues[45] reviewed 13 patients with acute displaced scaphoid fractures who had undergone internal fixation with Herbert screws via a retrograde approach. Radiographic union in was obtained in 12 (92%) of 13 in an average of 9.2 weeks. Inoue and Shionoya[13] prospectively studied 79 patients with acute scaphoid fractures. In this series, 39 patients chose conservative treatment and 40 chose internal fixation via a volar retrograde percutaneous approach using Herbert screws. The conservative group was managed with a short arm thumb spica cast. Union was achieved in 38 of 39 in the conservative group in an average of 9.7 weeks and in 40 of 40 patients in the surgical group in an average of 6 weeks. Average time for return to work was 10.2 weeks in the conservative group and 5.8 weeks in the surgical group.

Acutrak versus Herbert screws

Although there have been a number of biomechanical studies comparing the first generation Herbert screws to the second generation screws, there has been a relative paucity of clinical trials. Gregory and colleagues[46] compared 22 patients treated with Herbert screws and 23 patients treated with Acutrak screws for scaphoid nonunions and found no difference in union rate or time to union. Nineteen of 23 patients treated with Acutrak screws achieved union and 18 of 22 patients treated with Herbert screws achieved union. There was no difference in range of motion or pain between the 2 groups. Two patients from the Herbert group and 5 from the Acutrak group required screw removal because of hardware prominence. The difference in rate of screw removal was attributed to more complete visualization in the Herbert screw group and inappropriately long screw length in the Acutrak group.

SUMMARY

Scaphoid fractures carry significant long-term morbidity and short-term socioeconomic difficulty in the young and active patient population in which they most commonly occur. Treatment of scaphoid fractures has evolved from cast immobilization to open reduction internal fixation with K-wires, to internal fixation with traditional cancellous lag screws, to headless compression screws, and finally to specially designed headless, cannulated compression screws. Although cast immobilization results in high rates of radiographic union in nondisplaced scaphoid fractures, internal fixation has resulted in high rates of union in both nondisplaced and displaced fractures with the added benefits of early immobilization and return to work and sports. The development of percutaneous techniques has decreased perioperative morbidity and allowed faster recovery.

Multiple manufacturers are now offering headless compression screws for the internal fixation of scaphoid fractures. There are few studies directly comparing outcomes among the different screw manufacturers. The few biomechanical studies that exist demonstrate improved compression forces and load to failure for the newer generation of headless compression screws when compared with the traditional Herbert screw.

REFERENCES

1. Haisman JM, Rohde RS, Weiland AJ, et al. Acute fractures of the scaphoid. J Bone Joint Surg Am 2006;88(12):2750–8.
2. Chan KW, McAdams TR. Central screw placement in percutaneous screw scaphoid fixation: a cadaveric comparison of proximal and distal techniques. J Hand Surg Am 2004;29(1):74–9.
3. Soubeyrand M, Biau D, Mansour C, et al. Comparison of percutaneous dorsal versus volar fixation of scaphoid waist fractures using a computer model in cadavers. J Hand Surg Am 2009; 34(10):1838–44.
4. Streli R. [Percutaneous screwing of the navicular bone of the hand with a compression drill screw (a new method)]. Zentralbl Chir 1970;95:1060–78 [in German].
5. McQueen MM, Gelbke MK, Wakefield A, et al. Percutaneous screw fixation versus conservative treatment for fractures of the waist of the scaphoid:

6. Kozin SH. Incidence, mechanism, and natural history of scaphoid fractures. Hand Clin 2001; 17(4):515–24.
7. Geissler WB. Arthroscopic management of scaphoid fractures in athletes. Hand Clin 2009; 25(3):359–69.
8. Berger RA. The anatomy of the scaphoid. Hand Clin 2001;17(4):525–32.
9. Ring D. Nondisplaced scaphoid fractures: assessment and treatment. J Bone Joint Surg Am 2002; 84(1):144–5.
10. Adams JE, Steinmann SP. Acute scaphoid fractures. Orthop Clin North Am 2007;38(2):229–35, vi.
11. Ring D, Jupiter JB, Herndon JH. Acute fractures of the scaphoid. J Am Acad Orthop Surg 2000; 8(4):225–31.
12. Gellman H, Caputo RJ, Carter V, et al. Comparison of short and long thumb-spica casts for non-displaced fractures of the carpal scaphoid. J Bone Joint Surg Am 1989;71(3):354–7.
13. Inoue G, Shionoya K. Herbert screw fixation by limited access for acute fractures of the scaphoid. J Bone Joint Surg Br 1997;79(3):418–21.
14. Cooney WP. Herbert screw fixation of scaphoid fractures. J Bone Joint Surg Br 1998;80(1):181–2.
15. Cooney WP, Dobyns JH, Linscheid RL. Fractures of the scaphoid: a rational approach to management. Clin Orthop Relat Res 1980;149:90–7.
16. Capo JT, Orillaza NS Jr, Slade JF 3rd. Percutaneous management of scaphoid nonunions. Tech Hand Up Extrem Surg 2009;13(1):23–9.
17. Bedi A, Jebson PJ, Hayden RJ, et al. Internal fixation of acute, nondisplaced scaphoid waist fractures via a limited dorsal approach: an assessment of radiographic and functional outcomes. J Hand Surg Am 2007;32(3):326–33.
18. Bond CD, Shin AY, McBride MT, et al. Percutaneous screw fixation or cast immobilization for nondisplaced scaphoid fractures. J Bone Joint Surg Am 2001;83(4):483–8.
19. Shin AY, Hofmeister EP. Percutaneous fixation of stable scaphoid fractures. Tech Hand Up Extrem Surg 2004;8(2):87–94.
20. Cosio MQ, Camp RA. Percutaneous pinning of symptomatic scaphoid nonunions. J Hand Surg Am 1986;11(3):350–5.
21. Wozasek GE, Moser KD. Percutaneous screw fixation for fractures of the scaphoid. J Bone Joint Surg Br 1991;73(1):138–42.
22. Ledoux P, Chahidi N, Moermans JP, et al. Percutaneous Herbert screw osteosynthesis of the scaphoid bone. Acta Orthop Belg 1995;61(1):43–7.
23. Herbert TJ, Fisher WE. Management of the fractured scaphoid using a new bone screw. J Bone Joint Surg Br 1984;66(1):114–23.

a prospective randomised study. J Bone Joint Surg Br 2008;90(1):66–71.

24. Whipple TL. The role of arthroscopy in the treatment of intra-articular wrist fractures. Hand Clin 1995;11:13–8.

25. Slade JF 3rd, Jaskwhich D. Percutaneous fixation of scaphoid fractures. Hand Clin 2001;17(4):553–74.

26. Whipple TL. The role of arthroscopy in the treatment of scapholunate instability. Hand Clin 1995; 11(1):37–40.

27. Trumble TE, Clarke T, Kreder HJ. Non-union of the scaphoid. Treatment with cannulated screws compared with treatment with Herbert screws. J Bone Joint Surg Am 1996;78(12):1829–37.

28. Trumble TE, Gilbert M, Murray LW, et al. Displaced scaphoid fractures treated with open reduction and internal fixation with a cannulated screw. J Bone Joint Surg Am 2000;82(5):633–41.

29. Kozin SH. Internal fixation of scaphoid fractures. Hand Clin 1997;13(4):573–86.

30. Hausmann JT, Mayr W, Unger E, et al. Interfragmentary compression forces of scaphoid screws in a sawbone cylinder model. Injury 2007;38(7):763–8.

31. Toby EB, Butler TE, McCormack TJ, et al. A comparison of fixation screws for the scaphoid during application of cyclical bending loads. J Bone Joint Surg Am 1997;79(8):1190–7.

32. McCallister WV, Knight J, Kaliappan R, et al. Central placement of the screw in simulated fractures of the scaphoid waist: a biomechanical study. J Bone Joint Surg Am 2003;85(1):72–7.

33. Dodds SD, Panjabi MM, Slade JF 3rd. Screw fixation of scaphoid fractures: a biomechanical assessment of screw length and screw augmentation. J Hand Surg Am 2006;31(3):405–13.

34. Lo IK, King GJ, Milne AD, et al. A biomechanical analysis of intrascaphoid compression using the Herbert scaphoid screw system. An in vitro cadaveric study. J Hand Surg Br 1998; 23(2):209–13.

35. Adla DN, Kitsis C, Miles AW. Compression forces generated by Mini bone screws—a comparative study done on bone model. Injury 2005;36(1):65–70.

36. Beadel GP, Ferreira L, Johnson JA, et al. Interfragmentary compression across a simulated scaphoid fracture—analysis of 3 screws. J Hand Surg Am 2004;29(2):273–8.

37. Wheeler DL, McLoughlin SW. Biomechanical assessment of compression screws. Clin Orthop Relat Res 1998;350:237–45.

38. Newport ML, Williams CD, Bradley WD. Mechanical strength of scaphoid fixation. J Hand Surg Br 1996; 21(1):99–102.

39. Herbert TJ. Open volar repair of acute scaphoid fractures. Hand Clin 2001;17(4):589–99, viii.

40. Bond CD, Shin CA. Percutaneous cannulated screw fixation of acute scaphoid fractures. Tech Hand Up Extrem Surg 2000;4(2):81–7.

41. Adolfsson L, Lindau T, Arner M. Acutrak screw fixation versus cast immobilisation for undisplaced scaphoid waist fractures. J Hand Surg Br 2001;26(3):192–5.

42. Haddad FS, Goddard NJ. Acute percutaneous scaphoid fixation using a cannulated screw. Chir Main 1998;17(2):119–26.

43. Chen AC, Chao EK, Hung SS, et al. Percutaneous screw fixation for unstable scaphoid fractures. J Trauma 2005;59(1):184–7.

44. Rettig ME, Kozin SH, Cooney WP. Open reduction and internal fixation of acute displaced scaphoid waist fractures. J Hand Surg Am 2001;26(2):271–6.

45. Jeon IH, Oh CW, Park BC, et al. Minimal invasive percutaneous Herbert screw fixation in acute unstable scaphoid fracture. Hand Surg 2003;8(2): 213–8.

46. Gregory JJ, Mohil RS, Ng AB, et al. Comparison of Herbert and Acutrak screws in the treatment of scaphoid non-union and delayed union. Acta Orthop Belg 2008;74(6):761–5.

Intramedullary Fixation of Distal Radius Fractures

Kevin Harreld, MD, Zhongyu Li, MD, PhD*

KEYWORDS

- Distal radius fracture • Intramedullary fixation
- Minimally invasive

Colles first reported on distal radius fractures in 1814. Even then, he appreciated the ubiquitous nature of this injury, noting "I should consider this as by far the most common injury to which the wrist or carpal extremities of the radius and ulna are exposed."[1] Distal radius fractures remain a common occurrence today, with recent studies reporting an overall incidence of 125 per 10,000 Medicare beneficiaries.[2] Additionally, a prospective, multicenter, epidemiologic study estimated the incidence to be 36.8 out of 10,000 person-years in women and 9.0 out of 10,000 person-years in men aged more than 35 years.[3] The growth in the percentage of the population more than 65 years of age, in conjunction with an increased level of activity in elderly individuals, can be expected to result in ever increasing numbers of distal radius fractures in the future.[4]

A multitude of different techniques have been described for management of these fractures. Conservative measures include closed reduction and casting. However, malunion and resultant dysfunction remain a concern in the unstable or intraarticular fracture caused by either inadequate reduction or loss of reduction.[5] Surgical treatment options are varied and include percutaneous pinning,[6–8] bridging external fixation,[9–11] nonbridging external fixation,[12–15] and open reduction and internal fixation through a volar,[16–21] dorsal,[22–26] or combined[27] approach. Despite the multitude of studies dedicated to comparison of these techniques, a recent Cochrane review revealed insufficient evidence to recommend any one treatment over another.[28] Each treatment modality has its own inherent merit and disadvantages.

In recent years, the advent of the volar locking plate has brought about a general trend toward more aggressive fracture fixation, particularly in the elderly.[29] This trend is in large part because of the ability of locking-plate technology to impart sufficient stability to the fracture to enable range of motion at an earlier time point than previous methods of fixation.[30] This early range of motion is presumably responsible for the improved rate of functional recovery in the elderly age group, which was recently found to be comparable to younger adults aged 20 to 40 years.[19] However, the rise in use of volar plating has been associated with increased recognition of complications associated with this approach. Reported complications have included carpal tunnel syndrome[31]; flexor tendon injuries,[32] including flexor pollicis longus (FPL) rupture[33,34]; extensor tendon injuries,[16,35] including extensor pollicis longus (EPL) rupture[36,37]; and hardware failure with loss of reduction.[31]

Intramedullary nailing of the distal radius has recently been growing in popularity as a means to avoid the potential soft-tissue complications associated with volar plating, yet take advantage of the benefits of early range of motion afforded by locking technology.[38] The intramedullary implant most widely used in the United States is the Micronail (Wright Medical Technology, Inc, Arlington, TN, USA) (**Fig. 1**). It is a titanium alloy (Ti-6Al-4V ELI) implant designed to be inserted through the radial

Department of Orthopaedic Surgery, Wake Forest University School of Medicine, Medical Center Boulevard, Winston-Salem, NC 27157, USA
* Corresponding author.
E-mail address: zli@wfubmc.edu

Hand Clin 26 (2010) 363–372
doi:10.1016/j.hcl.2010.04.009

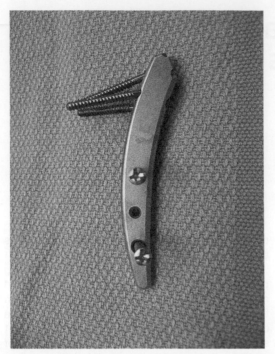

Fig. 1. Clinical photograph of the Micronail. The distal subchondral locking screws are purple and seen at the left of the image. The gold proximal interlocking screws are seen lying in their respective interlocking holes in the nail.

styloid and to rest completely within the confines of the intramedullary canal of the distal radius. Three 2.5-mm fixed angle locking screws are used to buttress the subchondral bone and secure the distal fragment to the implant. Two 2.7-mm cortex screws secure the nail to the shaft proximally.

Other designs for intramedullary fixation are also commercially available. The Targon DR (Aesculap, Tuttlingen, Germany) is primarily used in European centers. Like the Micronail, it resides completely within the intramedullary canal and is inserted through the radial styloid. The proximal interlocking screws, however, are inserted in a radial-to-ulnar rather than dorsal-to-volar direction. The Dorsal Nail Plate (Depuy, Warsaw, IN, USA) is a hybrid device, incorporating intramedullary and extramedullary components. It is inserted through a dorsal incision overlying Lister's tubercle. The implant is subsequently inserted into the medullary canal through a small corticotomy of the tubercle. The distal portion of the device is extramedullary, lying on the dorsal cortex of the distal radius in the floor of the third extensor compartment. The distal screws are placed dorsal to volar and are divergent in nature. Three proximal interlocking screws are placed through the same incision with the use of a targeting jig to rotationally lock the nail. The

WavEon WRx (Sonoma Orthopedic Products, Santa Rosa, CA, USA) is the latest product in this category to be developed. At the time of this article's publication it is not currently available in general distribution. This device is inserted through the radial styloid. However, it is unique in that the device is self-anchoring in the intramedullary canal. Two sets of grippers are expandable from the body of the implant, providing interference fit within the canal. As a result, no proximal interlocking screws are required. The authors have no personal experience with these other devices and there is limited published data available for these implants. Consequently, the following sections are primarily in reference to the Micronail, with outcomes of other implants reported as available.

ADVANTAGES

Proposed benefits of an intramedullary implant include biomechanical and soft-tissue advantages. Like most intramedullary nails, the procedure is minimally invasive in nature, requiring less exposure and soft-tissue dissection than standard plating techniques. The implant is inserted through a 2-cm incision over the radial styloid. Dorsal-to-volar interlocking screws are placed percutaneously or through a second 2-cm incisio proximally. Minimal soft-tissue disruption is required, resulting in less potential postoperative adhesion and less potential injury to neurovascular structures or tendons in the approach.[38] Theoretically, less soft-tissue disruption should result in less postoperative pain and improved ability to tolerate an accelerated postoperative therapy protocol. Additionally, as the implant resides completely within the confines of the intramedullary canal, there is less potential for tendon or soft-tissue irritation.[38] Ilyas and Thoder recently reported a series of 10 cases in which there was no incidence of tendon or soft-tissue irritation or need for hardware removal.[39]

Biomechanical advantages of the implant include the use of locking-screw technology to create a fixed-angle device, a divergent screw pattern in the distal fragment to provide improved subchondral support and resistance to collapse, and load sharing capabilities similar to other intramedullary implants. These features impart sufficient stability to the construct to allow supervised range of motion as soon as tolerated by patients[38] or as allowed by the surgeon.[39,40] In a recent cadaveric model, the Micronail was significantly stronger than nonlocked dorsal plating in both the load to yield 5 mm of fracture displacement and in ultimate load to failure.[41] Additionally, there was no significant difference between load to yield 5 mm of displacement, ultimate load to failure, or in bending rigidity between the Micronail and a volar locking plate. In this model, there were no cases of screw pull out or loosening in the distal fragment with use of the Micronail and no evidence of implant deformation. In all cases, the construct failed by either fracture proximally through the shaft screw holes or at the junction of the bone-cement mounting interface to the materials testing machine.[41]

DISADVANTAGES

Despite the noted advantages, the minimally invasive nature of the intramedullary implant does also result in some potential disadvantages. Indirect techniques of fracture reduction are requisite for this implant. Consequently, difficulty may be encountered when attempting to use the Micronail for a fracture that is not easily reduced in a closed or percutaneous fashion. The implant itself, unlike a volar plate, cannot be employed in fracture reduction. Once the distal locking screws are in place, further manipulation of the fracture is limited.[39] Thus, the fracture must be held in a reduced position throughout the case. If the canal is broached with the fracture malreduced, it will be impossible to anatomically reduce the fracture with the actual implant. Rather, the implant will follow the path of the broaches and stabilize the fracture in the malreduced position. Intramedullary nailing also has limited ability to control fractures with metaphyseal-diaphyseal extension and those with a coronal split.[38,39] Another concern relates to sagittal plane alignment. The radial-to-ulnar orientation of the distal screws limits the ability of the implant to facilitate and maintain fracture reduction in the sagittal plane.[39] With earlier versions of the Micronail instrumentation, there was some difficulty in assessing sagittal plane alignment during nail insertion because the overlying jig obscured imaging attempts in this plane.[40] A newer radiolucent design has helped overcome this limitation; however, correct sagittal plane alignment should still be established in initial reduction and broaching. Lastly, despite the design of the nail to reside completely within the intramedullary canal, placement of excessively long screws in the shaft or distal fragment may still result in soft-tissue irritation. Screw penetration into the radiocarpal or distal radioulnar joint is a possibility, but can be readily avoided with adequate fluoroscopic visualization.[39,40]

INDICATIONS/CONTRAINDICATIONS

Primary indications for intramedullary fixation include unstable extra-articular arbeitsgemeinschaft fur osteosynthesefragen (AO) type A fractures or AO type C1 fractures, in which there is a simple intraarticular pattern with large fragments conducive to closed or percutaneous reduction methods. Potential indications for intramedullary nailing include patients in whom minimal surgical dissection is desired, elderly patients with poor bone quality, polytrauma patients who require early mobilization, or fractures that have redisplaced with cast treatment.[38] Additionally, use of some intramedullary implants has recently expanded to include fixation following a corrective distal radius osteotomy in the management of malunions. However, application should be limited to extra-articular malunions and not be used for fixation of malunions requiring an intraarticular osteotomy.[42]

Contraindications include fractures in which there are multiple, small comminuted articular fragments.[38] Indications are expanding to include intraarticular fractures with a simple coronal split using a custom designed jig (Akihiro Maruo, MD, personal communication, 2009); however, the authors have no direct experience in using intramedullary implants for these fracture subtypes. Also, shear fracture patterns, such as volar or dorsal Barton's fractures, or other AO type B fracture patterns cannot be adequately buttressed by the intramedullary implant.[39,42] Additional contraindications include pediatric patients with open physes, fracture extension into the metaphyseal-diaphyseal bone, and open fractures.[38,43]

SURGICAL TECHNIQUE

Surgery may be performed under either regional or general anesthesia. Patients are positioned supine with the affected extremity placed laterally to rest on an arm table. Placement of the implant will require a limited radial and dorsal approach to the wrist. Use of a tourniquet will facilitate identification of critical neurovascular structures during the approach. Following establishment of a sterile surgical field, the first step is to verify that the fracture is amenable to closed or percutaneous reduction. It is critical to confirm that the fracture can be adequately reduced and held with traction or percutaneous joysticks before initiating the procedure. If difficulty is encountered in closed or percutaneous reduction, a limited open technique can be employed. A small incision is made at the eventual location of either the radial styloid incision or the dorsal wrist incision. Generally, if the dorsal wrist incision is cheated slightly proximally one can still insert the proximal interlocks through the nail and yet access the fracture site with a Freer elevator through the same incision. The authors are frequently able to overcome a difficult closed

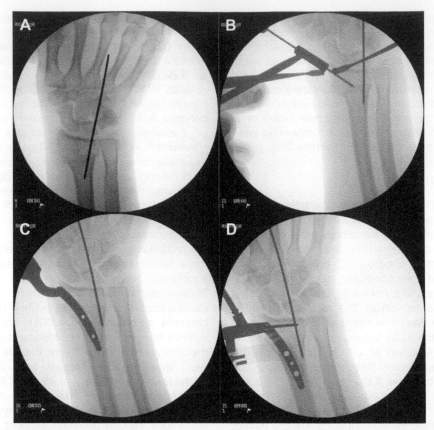

Fig. 2. (*A*) The initial K-wire is placed ulnar in the distal radius to avoid blocking the eventual path of the broach. (*B*) A guidewire is placed to establish the entry point for the nail. (*C*) The canal is sequentially broached. (*D*) The implant should be seated to a depth that ensures that the distal screws are within 2 mm of subchondral bone.

or percutaneous reduction with the use of a Freer elevator inserted into the fracture site through either or both of these incisions. Once intraoperative fluoroscopy confirms adequate reduction, a 0.062 in K-wire is placed dorsal to volar along the ulnar column to maintain reduction. Care must be taken to keep the K-wire out of the future path of the broaches and implant along the radial column (**Fig. 2**A). Once the fracture is reduced and temporarily stabilized, attention may be turned to beginning the surgical approach.

The primary landmark for the limited radial approach is the tip of the radial styloid. A 2-cm incision is made centered over the tip of the styloid. The structure most at risk with this approach is the superficial branch of the radial nerve, which will have arborized into several branches at this level. Great care should be taken to identify and protect all branches to avoid painful neuritis postoperatively. Dissection is carried down to identify the first and second dorsal extensor compartments. The 1, 2 intercompartmental supraretinacular artery and its venae comitantes may be used as a landmark to identify the

interval between these 2 compartments (**Fig. 3**). Avoid opening the compartments while subperiosteally elevating the first and second extensor compartments off the distal radius. The bare

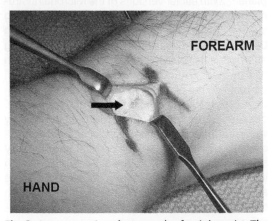

Fig. 3. Intraoperative photograph of a right wrist. The hand is at the bottom left of the frame and the forearm at the top right. The 1, 2 intercompartmental supraretinacular artery (*red arrow*) can be seen in the wound, delineating the plane for dissection.

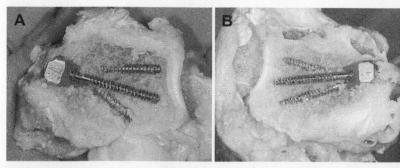

Fig. 4. (*A*) Cadaveric cross-section of a distal radius in which a Micronail has been inserted with the jig rotated off axis from the parallel plane. A resulting cortical perforation is evident. (*B*) When the jig is aligned parallel with the dorsal surface of the distal radius there is optimal screw spread in the volar to dorsal plane without cortical violation. *Reprinted from* Koman LA, editor. Wake Forest University School of Medicine Orthopaedic Manual. Winston Salem (NC): Orthopaedic Press; 2009. p. 9–10; with permission.

spot on the radial styloid between these 2 compartments will serve as the entry point for the intramedullary nail.

The entry hole for the implant is then established at the tip of the radial styloid at least 3 mm proximal to the articular surface. A guidewire is placed at the desired starting location (**Fig. 2**B). The cortex is then opened using a 6.1-mm cannulated drill over the guidewire. A starting awl is then passed into the intramedullary space across the reduced fracture. Care must be taken to stay radial in the canal, so as to not penetrate the ulnar cortex of the radial shaft with the starting awl. Sequential broaching is then performed until adequate fit of the canal is obtained (**Fig. 2**C). It is critical that fracture reduction be maintained during the entire

broaching process, because this determines the eventual path and location of the final implant. The desired fit is obtained when the broach does not spin in the canal with 2-finger pressure. Alternatively for patients with osteoporotic bone, the authors prefer to use the trial to enlarge the canal rather than the broach.

The appropriately sized implant is then attached to the insertion jig and advanced along the path of the broach until the tip of the nail is below the cortical surface of the radial styloid. It is critical to verify that the most distal locking screw will be extra-articular but within 2 mm of the articular surface to obtain maximum subchondral support (**Fig. 2**D). The jig should lie parallel to the dorsal surface of the forearm to ensure optimal length

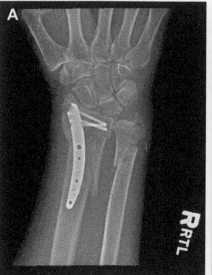
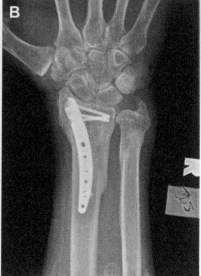

Fig. 5. (*A*) A 3-week follow-up of a distal radius fracture with metaphyseal extension treated with the long variety Micronail. (*B*) Subsequent 6-month follow-up of the same patient reveals union of the fracture.

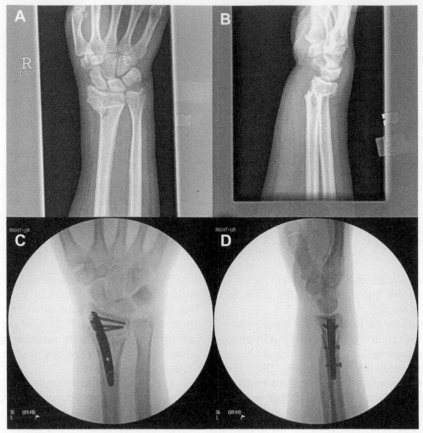

Fig. 6. (*A, B*) Anterior-posterior (AP) and lateral wrist radiographs of a 56-year-old woman who tripped over her dog and sustained a right-sided extra-articular distal radius fracture. (*C, D*) AP and lateral fluoroscopic images immediately following fixation with the Micronail.

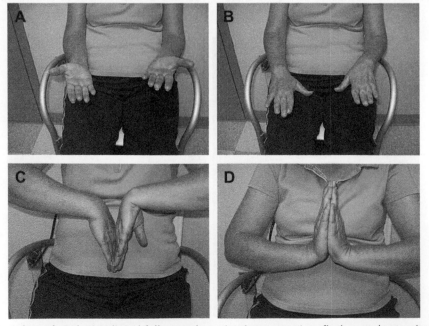

Fig. 7. Panels *A* through *D* depict clinical follow-up in supination, pronation, flexion, and extension of the fractured right wrist from **Fig. 6** at nearly 1.5 years.

Table 1
Outcomes following intramedullary fixation of distal radius fractures

Study	Age	F/U	Flex	Ext	Pro	Sup	Rad D	DASH	Grip %
Tan et al[44]	59 (31–83)	6 mo	58 (25–75)	73 (55–90)	87 (80–90)	78 (50–90)	22 (15–30)	8 (0–23)	80 (68–100)
Ilyas et al[39]	55 (20–79)	21 mo	67 (45–90)	71 (45–80)	85 (75–90)	82 (70–90)	22.5 (10–30)	8 (0–57)	91 (83–100)

All values represent mean with range in parentheses.
Abbreviations: DASH, Disabilities of the Arm, Shoulder, and Hand Score; Ext, wrist extension; Flex, wrist flexion; F/U, follow-up; Grip %, grip strength as percentage of contralateral uninjured hand; Pro, pronation; Rad D, Radial deviation; Sup, Supination.

and position of the distal locking screws. If the jig is rotated, the optimal screw length may not be obtained or the screws may exit the dorsal or volar cortex (**Fig. 4**). A long nail may be considered if there is extensive metaphyseal comminution (**Fig. 5**). The drill bit for the distal locking screws is then inserted by hand in the most distal screw guide of the jig. Three distal locking screws are placed in divergent paths using the external jig, which serves to lock the nail to the distal fragment and create a fixed-angle construct. In placing the distal locking screws, particular attention should be paid to the length of the screws to avoid penetration of the distal radioulnar joint (DRUJ). Some authors have recommended routinely downsizing from the measured length of the screws.[39]

The proximal interlocking screws are then placed dorsal to volar in the radial shaft using the jig. Prior to inserting the screws, fracture reduction should be confirmed again. Final adjustments in radial length can be made before insertion of the screws. Either a percutaneous or an open 2-cm incision may be used for screw placement. If an open approach is employed, the desired interval is between the second and third dorsal compartments. The screws should be placed in bicortically to ensure secure fixation. Final images should confirm adequate fracture reduction. If at any point in the procedure it appears that closed reduction is going to be unsuccessful or cannot be maintained, open reduction can generally be achieved with a Freer elevator through the radial styloid or dorsal incisions, as previously described. The skin is closed with nylon suture and a volar splint is applied.

OUTCOMES

Early experiences with use of the Micronail have been encouraging (**Figs. 6** and **7**). However, most reported results have been limited to preliminary reports of small case series with short-term follow-up.[38–40] In their initial description of the technique, Tan and colleagues[38] reported encouraging early clinical and radiographic results in an unpublished series of 15 subjects. Subsequently, Brooks and colleagues[40] further reviewed the results of a prospective analysis by Tan and colleagues[44] of 23 consecutive subjects at a 6-month follow-up interval. More recently, Ilyas and Thoder reported results with a minimum follow-up of 1 year in 10 subjects.[39] The clinical results of these studies are summarized in **Table 1**. Range of motion and grip strength are noted to be slightly superior in the study by Ilyas and Thoder, likely representing continued improvement of these parameters with the longer follow-up period of at least 1 year. Union rates have not been universally reported, but the results of Tan and colleagues note that complete reduction was maintained in all but 3 subjects. Two of these subjects had an AO type C2 fracture, with 1-mm settling of a die punch fragment in 1 subject and collapse at the fracture site resulting in 14° of dorsal angulation in the second. The third subject had an AO type B3 fracture and required conversion to a volar locking plate 2 weeks postoperatively. The investigators attribute this to diminished dorsal-volar divergence of the distal screws in the first-generation design of the device.[40] Ilyas and Thoder specifically avoided use of the Micronail for all AO type B and C2 or C3 fractures in their

Table 2
Radiographic results at final postoperative follow-up

Study	Age	F/U	VT (°)	RI (°)	RH (mm)	UV (mm)
Tan et al[44]	59 (31–83)	6 mo	4 (-14–14)	22 (12–25)	12 (9–16)	0.2 (-2.0–3.0)
Ilyas et al[39]	55 (20–79)	21 mo (12–28)	-2.2 (-20–10)	24 (21–34)	12 (11–14)	-0.6 (-1.0–2.0)

Abbreviations: F/U, follow-up; RH, radial height; RI, radial inclination; UV, ulnar variance; VT, volar tilt.

Table 3
Complications following intramedullary fixation of distal radius fractures

Study	Age	F/U	No	SBRN Neuritis	DRUJ Penetration	LOR	Tendon Irritation	Implant Removal
Tan et al[38]	—	—	15	3 (20%)	—	—	—	—
Tan et al[44]	59 (31–83)	6 mo	23	3 (13%)	—	3 (13%)	0	1
Ilyas et al[39]	55 (20–79)	21 mo (12–28)	10	2 (20%)	3 (30%)	2 (20%)	0	0

Abbreviations: F/U, follow-up; LOR, loss of reduction; No, number of patients included in report; SBRN, superficial branch of the radial nerve.

study. There were no cases of hardware failure or removal; however, they found loss of volar tilt in 2 subjects with AO type A3 fractures with extensive dorsal comminution. They concluded good outcomes could be obtained with intramedullary fixation of extra-articular and simple intraarticular fracture patterns.[39]

Radiographic outcomes of reported series are summarized in **Table 2**. Normal values for these parameters in the uninjured wrist have been reported to be 11.2° of volar tilt, 23.6° of radial inclination, 11.6 mm of radial height, and -0.6 mm of ulnar variance.[45] In both series, the Micronail was associated with restoration of all parameters to a normal value except for volar tilt, which remained on average more neutral to slightly dorsally tilted,[39,40] which is most likely caused by the linear design of the implant.

Reported complications have been similar across studies and are summarized in **Table 3**. Transient superficial radial nerve sensory neuritis has been reported in all series, ranging from 13% to 20% of cases, with symptoms universally resolving by 2 to 3 months.[38–40] Ilyas and Thoder reported 3 cases of screw penetration into the distal radioulnar joint with 1 resulting in late symptomatic DRUJ arthritis.[39] Loss of fracture reduction has occurred in AO type C2, B3, and A3 fractures as previously noted.[39,40] No cases of infection, hardware breakage, complex regional pain syndrome, tendon rupture, or irritation have been reported.

Recently, 2 reports following the use of the Targon DR nail have been published in the German literature.[46,47] Gradl and colleagues reported a 100% union rate in 103 subjects. The mean volar tilt was 2.05° and the radial length in relation to the distal ulna was 0.06 ± 0.05 mm from the contralateral uninjured side.[46] In a short-term retrospective review comparing the Targon DR with a volar locking plate, there was no significant difference between the 2 groups in range of motion at a mean follow-up of 5.0 months for the intramedullary group and 8.5 months for the plating group.[47]

However, radiographic evaluation demonstrated better restoration of volar tilt with a locking plate (mean 5.5°) than with the intramedullary implant (mean -2.5°). Restoration of radial length was more reliable in the intramedullary group. Subjects had a higher subjective satisfaction with the intramedullary implant, as demonstrated by Disabilities of the Arm, Shoulder, and Hand Score (DASH) scores. The investigators attributed this difference to the less invasive surgical approach used in the intramedullary group.[47]

SUMMARY

There are currently only a limited number of published reports regarding outcomes following intramedullary fixation of distal radius fractures. These reports are short-term in nature, but the available evidence suggests that satisfactory outcomes can be obtained with application of the Micronail for treatment of displaced extra-articular or simple intraarticular distal radius fractures. Caution should be advised in application to AO type A3 fractures with extensive dorsal comminution, and the implant should be avoided for complex intraarticular fractures or partial articular fractures with a volar or dorsal shear component. Particular care should be taken during the approach to avoid postoperative superficial radial sensory nerve neuritis and during placement of the distal screws to avoid penetration of the DRUJ. Midterm to long-term follow-up studies with larger numbers of subjects and prospective, randomized studies comparing intramedullary fixation to more traditional techniques are needed to better delineate the role of intramedullary fixation in care of these common injuries.

REFERENCES

1. Colles A. On the fracture of the carpal extremity of the radius. Edinburgh Med Sur J 1814;10:182.
2. Fanuele J, Koval KJ, Lurie J, et al. Distal radial fracture treatment: what you get may depend on your age and address. J Bone Joint Surg Am 2009;91(6):1313–9.

3. O'Neill TW, Cooper C, Finn JD, et al. Incidence of distal forearm fracture in British men and women. Osteoporos Int 2001;12(7):555–8.

4. Chen NC, Jupiter JB. Management of distal radial fractures. J Bone Joint Surg Am 2007; 89(9):2051–62.

5. Fernandez DL. Closed manipulation and casting of distal radius fractures. Hand Clin 2005;21(3):307–16.

6. Greatting MD, Bishop AT. Intrafocal (Kapandji) pinning of unstable fractures of the distal radius. Orthop Clin North Am 1993;24(2):301–7.

7. Rayhack JM. The history and evolution of percutaneous pinning of displaced distal radius fractures. Orthop Clin North Am 1993;24(2):287–300.

8. van Aaken J, Beaulieu JY, Fusetti C. Long-term outcomes of closed reduction and percutaneous pinning for the treatment of distal radius fractures. J Hand Surg Am 2009;34(5):963 [author reply 963–4].

9. Capo JT, Swan KG Jr, Tan V. External fixation techniques for distal radius fractures. Clin Orthop Relat Res 2006;445:30–41.

10. Sanders RA, Keppel FL, Waldrop JI. External fixation of distal radial fractures: results and complications. J Hand Surg Am 1991;16(3):385–91.

11. Hayes AJ, Duffy PJ, McQueen MM. Bridging and non-bridging external fixation in the treatment of unstable fractures of the distal radius: a retrospective study of 588 patients. Acta Orthop 2008; 79(4):540–7.

12. McQueen MM. Redisplaced unstable fractures of the distal radius. A randomised, prospective study of bridging versus non-bridging external fixation. J Bone Joint Surg Br 1998;80(4):665–9.

13. Yamako G, Ishii Y, Matsuda Y, et al. Biomechanical characteristics of nonbridging external fixators for distal radius fractures. J Hand Surg Am 2008;33(3):322–6.

14. Gradl G, Jupiter JB, Gierer P, et al. Fractures of the distal radius treated with a nonbridging external fixation technique using multiplanar k-wires. J Hand Surg Am 2005;30(5):960–8.

15. Mirza A, Jupiter JB, Reinhart MK, et al. Fractures of the distal radius treated with cross-pin fixation and a non-bridging external fixator, the CPX system: a preliminary report. J Hand Surg Am 2009;34(4):603–16.

16. Lee HC, Wong YS, Chan BK, et al. Fixation of distal radius fractures using AO titanium volar distal radius plate. Hand Surg 2003;8(1):7–15.

17. Orbay JL, Fernandez DL. Volar fixation for dorsally displaced fractures of the distal radius: a preliminary report. J Hand Surg Am 2002;27(2):205–15.

18. Orbay JL, Fernandez DL. Volar fixed-angle plate fixation for unstable distal radius fractures in the elderly patient. J Hand Surg Am 2004;29(1):96–102.

19. Chung KC, Squitieri L, Kim HM. Comparative outcomes study using the volar locking plating system for distal radius fractures in both young adults and adults older than 60 years. J Hand Surg Am 2008;33(6):809–19.

20. Ruch DS, Papadonikolakis A. Volar versus dorsal plating in the management of intra-articular distal radius fractures. J Hand Surg Am 2006;31(1):9–16.

21. Drobetz H, Kutscha-Lissberg E. Osteosynthesis of distal radial fractures with a volar locking screw plate system. Int Orthop 2003;27(1):1–6.

22. Ring D, Jupiter JB, Brennwald J, et al. Prospective multicenter trial of a plate for dorsal fixation of distal radius fractures. J Hand Surg Am 1997;22(5):777–84.

23. Rein S, Schikore H, Schneiders W, et al. Results of dorsal or volar plate fixation of AO type C3 distal radius fractures: a retrospective study. J Hand Surg Am 2007;32(7):954–61.

24. Suckel A, Spies S, Munst P. Dorsal (AO/ASIF) pi-plate osteosynthesis in the treatment of distal intraarticular radius fractures. J Hand Surg Br 2006;31(6):673–9.

25. Kamath AF, Zurakowski D, Day CS. Low-profile dorsal plating for dorsally angulated distal radius fractures: an outcomes study. J Hand Surg Am 2006;31(7):1061–7.

26. Rozental TD, Beredjiklian PK, Bozentka DJ. Functional outcome and complications following two types of dorsal plating for unstable fractures of the distal part of the radius. J Bone Joint Surg Am 2003;85(10):1956–60.

27. Ring D, Prommersberger K, Jupiter JB. Combined dorsal and volar plate fixation of complex fractures of the distal part of the radius. J Bone Joint Surg Am 2004;86(8):1646–52.

28. Handoll HH, Madhok R. Surgical interventions for treating distal radial fractures in adults. Cochrane Database Syst Rev 2003;3:CD003209.

29. Chung KC, Shauver MJ, Birkmeyer JD. Trends in the United States in the treatment of distal radial fractures in the elderly. J Bone Joint Surg Am 2009; 91(8):1868–73.

30. Ring D, Jupiter JB. Treatment of osteoporotic distal radius fractures. Osteoporos Int 2005; 16(Suppl 2):S80–4.

31. Berglund LM, Messer TM. Complications of volar plate fixation for managing distal radius fractures. J Am Acad Orthop Surg 2009;17(6):369–77.

32. Cross AW, Schmidt CC. Flexor tendon injuries following locked volar plating of distal radius fractures. J Hand Surg Am 2008;33(2):164–7.

33. Duncan SF, Weiland AJ. Delayed rupture of the flexor pollicis longus tendon after routine volar placement of a T-plate on the distal radius. Am J Orthop 2007;36(12):669–70.

34. Klug RA, Press CM, Gonzalez MH. Rupture of the flexor pollicis longus tendon after volar fixed-angle plating of a distal radius fracture: a case report. J Hand Surg Am 2007;32(7):984–8.

35. Arora R, Lutz M, Hennerbichler A, et al. Complications following internal fixation of unstable distal

radius fracture with a palmar locking-plate. J Orthop Trauma 2007;21(5):316–22.

36. Benson EC, DeCarvalho A, Mikola EA, et al. Two potential causes of EPL rupture after distal radius volar plate fixation. Clin Orthop Relat Res 2006; 451:218–22.

37. Al-Rashid M, Theivendran K, Craigen MA. Delayed ruptures of the extensor tendon secondary to the use of volar locking compression plates for distal radial fractures. J Bone Joint Surg Br 2006;88(12): 1610–2.

38. Tan V, Capo J, Warburton M. Distal radius fracture fixation with an intramedullary nail. Tech Hand Up Extrem Surg 2005;9(4):195–201.

39. Ilyas AM, Thoder JJ. Intramedullary fixation of displaced distal radius fractures: a preliminary report. J Hand Surg Am 2008;33(10):1706–15.

40. Brooks KR, Capo JT, Warburton M, et al. Internal fixation of distal radius fractures with novel intramedullary implants. Clin Orthop Relat Res 2006;445:42–50.

41. Capo JT, Kinchelow T, Brooks K, et al. Biomechanical stability of four fixation constructs for

distal radius fractures. Hand (N Y) 2009;4(3): 272–8.

42. Ilyas AM, Reish MW, Beg TM, et al. Treatment of distal radius malunions with an intramedullary nail. Tech Hand Up Extrem Surg 2009;13(1):30–3.

43. Ilyas AM. Intramedullary fixation of distal radius fractures. J Hand Surg Am 2009;34(2):341–6.

44. Tan V, Capo J, Warburton M. Minimally invasive distal radius fracture fixation with an intramedullary nail. Annual Meeting of the American Society for Surgery of the Hand (ASSH). San Antonio (TX), September 22, 2005.

45. Medoff RJ. Essential radiographic evaluation for distal radius fractures. Hand Clin 2005;21(3):279–88.

46. Gradl G, Wendt M, Gierer P, et al. [Fixation of distal radial fractures with the Targon DR nail]. Oper Orthop Traumatol 2009;21(4-5):472–83 [in German].

47. Lerch S, Sextro HG, Wilken F, et al. [Clinical and radiological results after distal radius fracture: intramedullary locking nail versus volar locking plate osteosynthesis]. Z Orthop Unfall 2009; 147(5):547–52 [in German].

Variable-Angle Locking Screw Volar Plating of Distal Radius Fractures

Jung H. Park, MD[a], Jennifer Hagopian, MS, ATC[b], Asif M. Ilyas, MD[c,d],*

KEYWORDS

- Radius fracture • Variable-angle locking plate
- Volar plate • ORIF • Aptus • Variax • Viper

Distal radius fractures are among the most common fractures observed in emergency rooms and constitute up to 15% of all extremity fractures.[1,2] As life expectancies increase and the prevalence of osteopenia climbs, it is estimated that the incidence of these injuries will continue to increase over the next decade.[1,2] Although once believed that Colles fractures do well nonsurgically in all cases, it is now understood that anatomic restoration of the distal radius and its articular surface is central to avoiding the development of post-traumatic arthritis, wrist instability, and painful range of motion.[3–5] Treatment options for distal radius fractures vary widely from closed reduction and casting, percutaneous pinning or external fixation, and open reduction and internal fixation (ORIF). Although closed reduction and casting remain viable options with satisfactory long-term outcomes in certain fracture characteristics,[5–8] the role for ORIF has grown with its ability to more reliably restore wrist anatomy, minimize immobilization, and establish acceptable outcomes.[9–14] ORIF options include volar plating, radial plating, dorsal plating, fragment specific fixation, and intramedullary nailing. In recent years, volar locked plating has grown in popularity due to its consistent surgical approach, capacity to provide stable fixation of periarticular fractures despite osteopenia or comminution, and ability to facilitate early motion and rehabilitation.[10,11] More recently, variable-angle locking screw volar plates have become available providing greater versatility with plate and screw fixation for the management of distal radius fractures (**Fig. 1**).

APPLIED ANATOMY OF THE DISTAL RADIUS

The distal radius has a biconcave distal articular surface that articulates with the scaphoid and lunate carpal bones. Along its ulnar border is the sigmoid notch, which articulates with the ulnar head. The scaphoid fossa is triangular in shape, while the lunate fossa is oval shaped. The radius of curvature of the sigmoid notch is usually larger than that of the ulnar head to allow translation and rotation of the distal radioulnar joint (DRUJ). Restoration of the articular congruency has been proposed as the most important single factor in achieving a good clinical outcome.[3,4,15,16] The metaphysis flares both in anteroposterior and lateral planes, and the thinnest cortical bone is observed along the dorsal and radial aspects,

[a] Department of Orthopaedic Surgery, Temple University Hospital, 3401 North Broad Street, Philadelphia, PA 19140, USA
[b] Temple Hand Center, Temple University Hospital, 3401 North Broad Street, Philadelphia, PA 19140, USA
[c] Hand & Wrist Service, Rothman Institute, 925 Chestnut Street, Philadelphia, PA 19107, USA
[d] Orthopaedic Surgery, Thomas Jefferson University Hospital, 111 South 11th Street, Philadelphia, PA 19107, USA
* Corresponding author. Orthopaedic Surgery, Thomas Jefferson University Hospital, 111 South 11th Street, Philadelphia, PA 19107.
E-mail address: aimd2001@yahoo.com

Hand Clin 26 (2010) 373–380
doi:10.1016/j.hcl.2010.04.003
0749-0712/10/$ – see front matter © 2010 Elsevier Inc. All rights reserved.

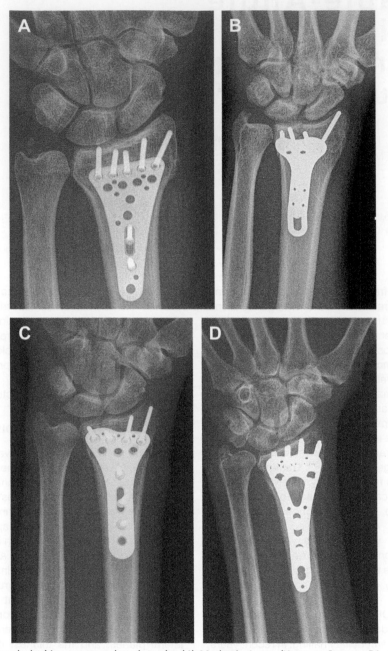

Fig. 1. Variable-angle locking screw volar plates by (*A*) Medartis Aptus (Kennett Square, PA, USA), (*B*) Trimed Volar Bearing Plate (Valencia, CA, USA), (*C*) Stryker Variax (Mahwah, NJ, USA), and (*D*) Synthes 2.4 mm Variable-Angle LCP Two-Column Volar Plate (Paoli, PA, USA).

hence the most common direction of collapse with most distal radius fractures. On the other hand, the strongest cortical bone, even in osteoporotic bones, is observed along the volar cortex under the lunate facet, which may contribute to the success in volar fixation technique.[10,11]

In treating distal radius fractures, articular congruency, volar tilt, radial inclination and height must be restored to avoid radiocarpal arthritis,

instability, and impingement causing painful range of motion.[3,4] Understanding of the normal anatomy of the distal radius is paramount in successful treatment of these injuries. Normal radiographic findings of the distal radius include average radial inclination of 23°, radial height of 11 mm, and volar tilt of 11°. Although there are no universally accepted postreduction parameters, commonly accepted values include: radial shortening less than 5 mm, radial inclination greater than 15°, between 15° dorsal and 20° volar tilt, and less than 2 mm of articular step off.[12] Beyond radiographic measurements, several additional variables also can be considered when determining whether a distal radius fracture may require an ORIF, including patient variables, associated injuries, and independent risk factors for fracture instability.

PLATING OPTIONS FOR THE DISTAL RADIUS

ORIF of distal radius fractures can be achieved through various surgical approaches dictated by surgeon preferences, fracture characteristics, and the needs of the selected implant. Plating options include dorsal plates, volar plates, and radial plates. Dorsal plates have enjoyed good success managing unstable distal radius fractures, particularly with dorsal angulation and comminution, but their proximity to the extensor tendons poses the potential for higher incidence of soft tissue complications including tendon adherence, tenosynovitis, and attritional rupture.[17,18] In contrast, volar plates have experienced good clinical outcomes along with an improved soft tissue profile.[9–12,19,20] Radial plates are effective in restoring radial height and augmenting fixation of unstable fractures.

VOLAR PLATES

There are numerous volar plates available for the management of distal radius fractures in the United States. They can be categorized as nonlocking, fixed-angle locking, and the more recent variable-angle locking plates. The conventional nonlocking plates rely on plate–bone interface and bicortical screw purchase for secure fixation. In osteoporotic bone and in severely comminuted fractures, however, the screws are prone to toggle and back out, risking loss of fracture reduction. This led to the introduction of fixed-angle volar plates, either one-piece or modular. Avanta introduced a one-piece blade plate that is anatomically shaped to restore the normal 12° volar tilt and 22° radial inclination. The tines are part of the plate, and they provide subchondral support. The lengths of the tines are pre-determined by the plate, however, and with the development of the modular fixed-angle plates that allow different length of each screw or peg, its popularity has declined.

Most modular fixed-angle locking volar plates have predetermined volar tilt and radial inclination designed into the plate, and the direction of the distal locking screws is therefore guided by the plate design. In most implants, distal locking is

available with fully and partially threaded screws or smooth pegs. The purposed advantage of smooth pegs is to minimize extensor tendon irritation, while still providing subchondral support when bicortical purchase is established. Biomechanical studies using screws versus pegs, however, showed that constructs with locking screws were significantly stronger than constructs with locking smooth pegs.[21] Because the direction of the distal screws ultimately is determined by the position of the plate, it is critical to optimize fracture reduction and plate position before screw placement to avoid inappropriate screw placement. There is abundant support in the literature for the use of fixed-angle locking volar plates demonstrating strong clinical outcomes, maintenance of anatomic reduction, and facilitation of early rehabilitation.[10–13]

Newer locking technology has resulted in the development of variable-angle locking screws with a range of motion up to 30° to 40° of angular variability between the plate and the locking screw. This increased versatility potentially allows more flexibility in both plate and screw placement. Several companies are currently manufacturing variable-angle locking volar plates. This article will review five such implants: Aptus (Medartis, Kenneth Square, PA, USA), Variax (Stryker, Mahwah, NJ, USA), Volar Bearing plate (Trimed, Valencia, CA, USA), 2.4 mm Variable-Angle LCP Two-Column Volar Plate (Synthes, Paoli, PA, USA), and Viper (Integra LifeSciences, Plainsboro, NJ, USA). The design and product features will be briefly reviewed in the following section.

Integra

Integra LifeSciences Viper with VALT (Variable-Angle Locking Technology) is an anatomic, side-specific titanium plate that allows a total of 40° of variable-angle screw placement before locking onto the plate. The locking mechanism is on the screw head and not on the plate; therefore, the screw can be seated onto the plate and lag large dorsal fragments before locking. Once satisfied with the angle of the distal screw position, the VALT key is used to turn the hub on the screw head 180° clockwise, while holding the screw stationary with the hold placement driver. This allows the hub on the screw head to turn independently and lock onto the plate. The cortical screws for the shaft are 3.5 mm, while the distal locking screws are 2.7 mm in core diameter, self-tapping and are available in 2 mm increments from 10 mm to 24 mm. There are two rows for distal screw fixation for a total of six screws, while there are four or six holes for cortical fixation.

Medartis Aptus

The Medartis Aptus 2.5 is a titanium, low-profile, side-specific, anatomically shaped plate (**Fig. 2**) that use 2.5 mm locking screws with a variable angle of plus or minus15° (**Fig. 3**). The locking mechanism is based on spherical three-point wedge locking (TriLock) that can be relocked up to three times. The locking screws are self-tapping yet have a smooth tip to prevent irritation of extensor tendons when bicortical fixation is achieved. A free drill guide is used to fit into the screw hole in the plate to confirm a variable angle within 15°. Locking screws are available in 2 mm increments from 8 mm to 34 mm. The plate has two rows of distal locking fixation and is available in narrow (22 mm) and regular (28 mm) for a total of seven to nine distal holes. K-wire holes are available in the plate for temporary fixation of the plate to bone. Plate length varies from 32 mm to up to 95 mm. Both the locking and nonlocking screws are 2.5 mm and similarly both use a 2.0 mm drill bit.

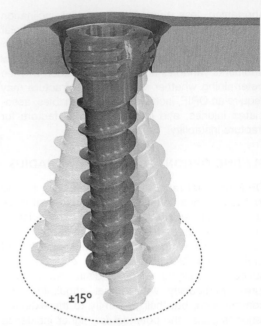

±15°

Fig. 3. Aptus Medartis locking screw illustrating the ±15° range of locking angles.

Either 2.5 mm screw can be placed in any hole in the plate including distally or proximally into the shaft.

Stryker Variax

The Stryker Variax plates are titanium plates that have undergone type 2 anodization treatment to improve tissue gliding and prevent adhesion formation. The polyaxial drill guide allows toggle within a 30° cone for each screw hole. Locking pegs are available in 2.0 mm diameter and locking screws in 2.3 mm and 2.7 mm diameters. The patented SmartLock locking is a one-step mechanism that relies on threads on the underside of the screw head to engage with the circular lip of the screw hole. The screw tip is blunt to allow bicortical fixation without extensor tendon irritation. Universal as well as side-specific anatomic plates are available. Anatomic plates are available in narrow and standard width and standard and long versions. There are two rows of distal locking holes for a total of five screw holes in narrow plates and seven holes in standard plates. Fixed-angle drill guide is also available for predetermined angles for the distal locking screws.

Synthes 2.4 Variable-Angle LCP

The Synthes 2.4 variable-angle LCP distal radius system is an anatomically designed plate. Screws can be locked within a 30° cone around the central axis of the plate. There are four columns of threads

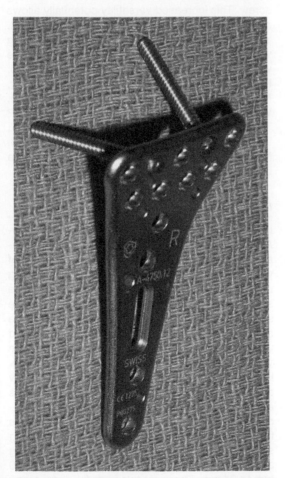

Fig. 2. Aptus Medartis variable-angle locking screw volar plate with distal subchondral screws placed at various angles.

in the screw holes allowing a four-point locking fixation. The two column volar plates have six to seven distal holes, while the extra-articular plate offers four to five holes. The proximal shaft features the combihole, which allows locking or nonlocking fixation, and plates are available in two-, three-, or four-shaft holes. The drill guide for the distal row is funnel shaped to allow drilling at variable angles. A 1.2 Nm torque limiting attachment for the screwdriver is provided with the system to avoid over-tightening upon final locking of the variable-angle screw. The screws are self-tapping tips and are available in 2 mm increments from 8 mm to 30 mm in length. Cortex screws are 2.4 mm or 2.7 mm in diameter and may be placed in any part of the combihole.

Trimed

The Trimed volar bearing plates are anatomic, side-specific plates made of stainless steel and available in standard and wide versions with the number of distal holes ranging from six to eight holes in two rows. Smooth pegs and threaded screws are available in 14 mm to 28 mm. The drill guide can be locked into the plate within 18° around a predetermined central angle. Length measurement can be estimated with the zebra striped K-wire with 5 mm increments or directly with a depth gauge after drill guide removal. The locking mechanism relies on four-point threaded ball-bearing fixation, which enlarges and engage when the tapered screw head is fully seated. The screw can be locked and unlocked up to five times.

OUTCOMES

To evaluate the efficacy of variable-angle volar locking plates for the management of unstable and displaced distal radius fractures, all consecutive patients treated over a 1-year period with an Aptus plate with a minimum follow-up of 6 months were retrospectively reviewed.

Methods

Between July 2008 and June 2009, 23 consecutive patients were treated with a Medartis Aptus plate. With a minimum of 6 months of follow-up, 20 patients were available for final review. There were 14 females and 6 males. The average patient age was 48 years (range 18 to 78 years). Fracture types included four arbeitsgemeinschaft für osteosynthesefragen (AO) type A (three A3, one A2), two AO type B (two B2), and 14 AO type C (five C1, four C2, five C3).

All fractures were reduced and internally fixed through the volar trans-FCR approach. A standardized postoperative rehabilitation was followed. Following surgery, all patients were discharged home with a volar plaster splint, and finger range of motion was encouraged. At 2 weeks postoperatively, the splint and sutures were removed, and a removable prefabricated splint was provided and physical therapy initiated. By 12 weeks postoperatively, all activity restrictions were removed. Patients were evaluated at 2, 6, 12, and 24 weeks postoperatively. Final study parameters included radiographic evidence of fracture union, hardware status, range of motion, the Disabilities of Arm, Shoulder, and Hand (DASH) score, and review of complications.

Technique

After administration of general anesthesia or application of a regional block, the injured extremity is prepared and draped across a hand table. Fluoroscopy is used throughout the operation to visualize the distal radius fracture (**Fig. 4**A). A trans-FCR approach is used to access the volar surface of the distal radius. The thumb and finger flexor tendons are retracted ulnarly, and the pronator quadratus is raised subperiosteally along its radial border and retracted ulnarly. The fracture is reduced under direct visualization and temporarily fixed with k-wires (see **Fig. 4**B). The goal is to restore volar tilt, radial height, radial inclination, ulnar variance, and articular alignment. A volar plate is applied to the reduced fracture and also temporarily transfixed with k-wires until satisfied with position of the plate. The plate initially is fixed to the shaft through the sliding hole. Distally, subchondral screws are placed beginning with non-locking screws to help further reduce the distal radial fragment and dial in additional volar tilt. Alternatively, the plate can be applied to the distal fragment first with locking screws followed by reduction of the plate to the shaft proximally (see **Fig. 4**C, D). In this fashion, the plate can be used to help restore volar tilt, radial height, inclination, and ulnar variance. Distally, variable-angle locking screws are used to strategically fix screws within the various articular fragments while diligently avoiding placement of screws in the radiocarpal and distal radioulnar joints. Final radiographs are scrutinized to confirm that the fracture is well reduced, the articular surfaces restored, and that the screws are not in the joint or too proud dorsally (see **Fig. 4**E). Postoperatively, the wrist is placed in a plaster volar splint with the elbow and fingers free. Finger range of motion is encouraged immediately after surgery. At the 2-week postoperative visit, the splint and dressings are removed, a removable splint fashioned, and range of motion

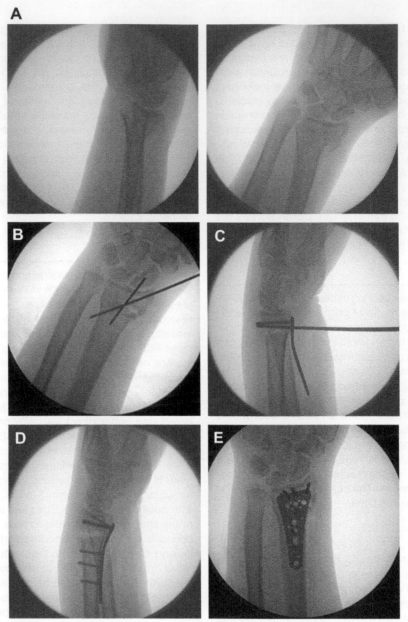

Fig. 4. Intraoperatively, (*A*) prereduction fluoroscopic images were reviewed, (*B*) fracture reduced and provisionally fixed with k-wires. (*C*) The volar plate is fixed distally with subchondral locking screws and (*D*) reduced proximally with the shaft screw to dial in additional volar tilt. (*E*) Final fluoroscopic views are reviewed to assess for quality of fracture reduction and position of the hardware.

exercises initiated under the supervision of a therapist. All restrictions are removed by the 12-week postoperative visit.

RESULTS

The average final follow-up time was 8 months (range, 6 to 11 months). All fractures healed uneventfully, with bridging callus evident in every case by the 12-week visit, except for one AO type A3 patient who required bone stimulator with eventual radiographic evidence of healing with bridging callus obtained by week 24. Further radiographic evaluation identified a final average volar tilt of 5.9° (range -2 to 16), radial height of 9.9 mm (range 7 to 13), radial inclination of 20.2° (range of 15 to 25), and ulnar variance of -0.75 mm (range of -3 to +1). Upon comparison of final follow-up radiographs to the initial postoperative images from day of surgery, no loss of reduction was identified in any case except for one where there was residual loss of articular alignment that required removal of hardware (AO type B2). In no case was there a failure of hardware, in particular, no loss of position or alignment of the variable-angle locking screws.

On final physical examination, the average wrist flexion was 80.0° (range 60° to 90°), extension 80.7° (range 70° to 90°), radial deviation 16.4° (range 5° to 35°), ulnar deviation 33.6° (range 30° to 45°), supination 78.6° (range 45° to 90°), and pronation 74.3° (range 30° to 90°). The average grip strength at final follow-up, as a percentage of their uninvolved contralateral extremity, was 83.3%. The average DASH score was 11.7 (range 1 to 30). There were no cases of soft tissue injuries, including nerve or tendon injuries.

DISCUSSION

Due to their relatively recent introduction, data concerning biomechanical and functional outcome of variable-angle volar locking plates in the literature are limited. Hoffmeier and colleagues studied the biomechanical strength of different variable-angle volar locking plates. In static loading, an increase of the screw-locking angle was associated with a reduction in ultimate and fatigue strength with the Palmar 2.7 and Viper locking interfaces, while not observed in the Variax system. During dynamic loading, however, decrease in locking strength was observed with the Variax, while not influenced in the Palmar 2.7.[22] Weninger and colleagues studied the biomechanical strength of an additional shaft screw (four shaft screws vs three) in a sawbone model using the Medartis Aptus plate. They found superior mechanical properties in the group with the additional protection screw, demonstrating the importance of the shaft screws in the overall mechanical property of these plates.[23]

Mehling and colleagues,[24] Vlcek and colleagues,[25] and Figl and colleagues[26] independently reported their experience using Medartis Aptus volar plate. Figl and colleagues reported the longest follow-up study using this system. In their 12-month outcome study, they showed that bone healing occurred in all 80 patients; 75% of patients had no radial shortening, while the remaining 25% experienced shortening of 1 mm to 3 mm. The average volar tilt was 6°, while average the radial inclination was 22°. The mean DASH score was 25 points; grip strength was 65%, and the greatest disparity in range of motion was seen in flexion/extension, which averaged to loss of 21% of contralateral side.[26] Mehling and colleagues[24] reported clinical results with a DASH score of 14 points and average grip strength of 85% in their 9-month outcome study.

These authors concluded that the Medartis Aptus system allows anatomic reduction with low complication rates, including low rates of secondary loss of reduction.[24–26]

Wong and colleagues reported their prospective cohort series with the Styker Variax plate in 35 patients with dorsally displaced distal radius fractures. The average healing time was 7 weeks, and two patients had complications. One patient had early loss of reduction, and one patient developed complex regional pain syndrome. The average Mayo Clinic wrist score at final follow up was 90, with 32 of 35 patients reporting good or excellent results.[27] Hakimi and colleagues reported their 12-month follow-up of a prospective cohort study using the Stryker Variax plate and found similar radiographic and clinical outcomes when compared with the uniaxial locking plate group. However, the variable-angle locking plate group required 58 seconds longer intraoperative fluoroscopy time.[28] There are also comparative studies of volar variable-angle fixed plates (Medartis Aptus) versus an intramedullary nail (Targon).[29] Lersh and colleagues reported similar range of motion between the two groups. On radiographic analysis, however, volar tilt was better achieved in the plating group (-2.5° vs 5.5°), while radial height was better restored in the intramedullary nail group. Most significantly, patients in the intramedullary nail group reported higher subjective satisfaction DASH scores (14 vs 23), which the authors attributed to the less-invasive surgical approach.[29]

SUMMARY

Volar locking plates, and most recently variable-angle locking screw volar locking plates, are growing in popularity in the treatment of displaced unstable distal radius fractures. The appeal of the variable-angle locking plate lies in the increased versatility for fracture fixation offered to the surgeon. Although the literature is limited, early biomechanical and clinical studies point to continued success of these new implants. The authors' experience with the Medartis Aptus plate provides strong support for our opinion. The authors observed acceptable fracture reduction, healing, and patient outcome with minimal complications and no loss of position of the variable-angle locking screw.

REFERENCES

1. Ismail AA, Pye SR, Cockerill WC, et al. Incidence of limb fracture across Europe: results from the European Prospective Osteoporosis Study (EPOS). Osteoporos Int 2002;13(7):565–71.

2. Chung KC, Spilson SV. The frequency and epidemiology of hand and forearm fractures in the United States. J Hand Surg Am 2001;26(5):908–15.

3. Trumble TE, Schmitt SR, Vedder NB. Factors affecting functional outcome of displaced intra-articular distal radius fractures. J Hand Surg Am 1994; 19(2):325–40.

4. Forward DP, Davis TR, Sithole JS. Do young patients with malunited fractures of the distal radius inevitably develop symptomatic post-traumatic osteoarthritis? J Bone Joint Surg Br 2008;90(5):629–37.

5. Catalano LW 3rd, Cole RJ, Gelberman RH, et al. Displaced intra-articular fractures of the distal aspect of the radius. Long-term results in young adults after open reduction and internal fixation. J Bone Joint Surg Am 1997;79(9):1290–302.

6. Synn AJ, Makhni EC, Makhni MC, et al. Distal radius fractures in older patients: is anatomic reduction necessary? Clin Orthop Relat Res 2009;467(6): 1612–20.

7. Arora R, Gabl M, Gschwentner M, et al. A comparative study of clinical and radiologic outcomes of unstable colles type distal radius fractures in patients older than 70 years: nonoperative treatment versus volar locking plating. J Orthop Trauma 2009; 23(4):237–42.

8. Rohde G, Haugeberg G, Mengshoel AM, et al. No long-term impact of low-energy distal radius fracture on health-related quality of life and global quality of life: a case–control study. BMC Musculoskelet Disord 2009;10:106.

9. Koenig KM, Davis GC, Grove MR, et al. Is early internal fixation preferred to cast treatment for well-reduced unstable distal radial fractures? J Bone Joint Surg Am 2009;91(9):2086–93.

10. Orbay JL, Fernandez DL. Volar fixed-angle plate fixation for unstable distal radius fractures in the elderly patient. J Hand Surg Am 2004;29(1):96–102.

11. Mudgal CS, Jupiter JB. Plate fixation of osteoporotic fractures of the distal radius. J Orthop Trauma 2008; 22(Suppl 8):S106–15.

12. Nana AD, Joshi A, Lichtman DM. Plating of the distal radius. J Am Acad Orthop Surg 2005;13(3):159–71.

13. Jupiter JB, Marent-Huber M, LCP Study Group. Operative management of distal radial fractures with 2.4 millimeter locking plates. A multicenter prospective case series. J Bone Joint Surg Am 2009;91(1):55–65.

14. Smith D, Henry M. Volar fixed-angle plating of the distal radius. J Am Acad Orthop Surg 2005;13(1): 28–36.

15. Vasenius J. Operative treatment of distal radius fractures. Scand J Surg 2008;97(4):290–6.

16. Rikli DA, Regazzoni P, Babst R. Dorsal double plating for fractures of the distal radius—a biomechanical concept and clinical experience. Zentralbl Chir 2003;128(12):1003–7.

17. Grewal R, Perey B, Wilmink M, et al. A randomized prospective study on the treatment of intra-articular distal radius fractures: open reduction and internal fixation with dorsal plating versus mini open reduction, percutaneous fixation, and external fixation. J Hand Surg Am 2005;30(4):764–72.

18. Berglund L, Messer T. Complications of volar plate fixation for managing distal radius fractures. J Am Acad Orthop Surg 2009;17:369–77.

19. Protopsaltis TS, Ruch DS. Volar fixed-angle plating of the distal radius. J Hand Surg Am 2008;33(6): 958–65.

20. Kandemir U, Matityahu A, Desai R, et al. Does a volar locking plate provide equivalent stability as a dorsal nonlocking plate in a dorsally comminuted distal radius fracture? a biomechanical study. J Orthop Trauma 2008;22(9):605–10.

21. Martineau PA, Waitayawinyu T, Malone KJ, et al. Volar plating of AO C3 distal radius fractures: biomechanical evaluation of locking screw and locking smooth peg configurations. J Hand Surg Am 2008; 33(6):827–34.

22. Hoffmeier KL, Hofmann GO, Mückley T. The strength of polyaxial locking interfaces of distal radius plates. Clin Biomech 2009;24(8):637–41.

23. Weninger P, Schueller M, Drobetz H, et al. Influence of an additional locking screw on fracture reduction after volar fixed-angle plating-introduction of the protection screw in an extra-articular distal radius fracture model. J Trauma 2009;67(4):746–51.

24. Mehling I, Meier M, Schlör U, et al. Multidirectional palmar fixed-angle plate fixation for unstable distal radius. Handchir Mikrochir Plast Chir 2007;39(1): 29–33.

25. Vlcek M, Visna P. Six-month functional and X-ray outcomes of distal radius fractures managed using multidirectional locking plates. Rozhl Chir 2008; 87(9):486–92.

26. Figl M, Weninger P, Liska M, et al. Volar fixed-angle plate osteosynthesis of unstable distal radius fractures: 12-months results. Arch Orthop Trauma Surg 2009;129:661–9.

27. Wong TC, Yeung CC, Chiu Y, et al. Palmar fixation of dorsally displaced distal radius fractures using locking plates with Smartlock locking screws. J Hand Surg Eur Vol 2009;34(2):173–8.

28. Hakimi M, Jungbluth P, Gehrmann S, et al. Unidirectional versus multidirectional palmar locking osteosynthesis of unstable distal radius fractures: comparative analysis with LDR 2.4 mm versus 2.7 mm matrix-smartlock. Unfallchirurgie 2010; 113(3):210–6.

29. Lerch S, Sextro HG, Wilken F, et al. Clinical and radiological results after distal radius fracture: intramedullary locking nail versus volar locking plate osteosynthesis. Z Orthop Unfall 2009;147(5): 547–52.

Nonbridging External Fixation of Distal Radius Fractures

Matthew D. Eichenbaum, MD, Eon K. Shin, MD*

KEYWORDS

- Distal radius fracture • Nonbridging external fixation
- Malunion • Osteoporosis

As befits the most common fracture site in the upper extremity, the distal radius continues to be a topic of much clinical and scholarly discourse.[1] Accounting for one-sixth of all fractures treated in emergency departments and the most common fracture of any type in the adult population, fractures of the distal radius and their management continue to be a prime concern for general orthopedists and hand surgeons alike.[2] Awareness of the potential pitfalls associated with treating these injuries and identification of poorer than expected results from simple immobilization have spurred surgical and technologic advancements, thereby improving the treatment of distal radius injuries.

The traditional treatment for several decades after Abraham Colles' 1814 description of the distal radius fracture pattern, which now bears his name, consisted simply of cast immobilization alone.[3,4] Recognition that unstable distal radius fractures treated solely with cast immobilization are at risk for fragment collapse, fracture malunion, and possible disability prompted the evolution of closed and open reduction techniques in conjunction with various forms of external and internal fixation.[5-13] The expected growth of an aging adult population that lives longer and more actively predicts an increase in the number of osteoporotic fractures, a category that includes fractures of the distal radius.[14] Epidemiologic data suggest that 1 of every 10 white women aged 65 years old in the United States will sustain a fracture of the distal radius during her remaining lifetime.[15]

Recent trends have shown an increase in the use of internal fixation for surgical management of distal radius fractures after the introduction of the first volar locking plate system in 2000.[7,16-18] Despite the recognized growth of internal fixation, external fixation has maintained a role in the treatment of distal radius fractures because of its relative ease in application, versatility in use, and reduced effects on the pericarpal soft tissues.[19] Procedural and technologic advancements now permit nonbridging external fixation with fixator pins placed directly into distal radius fragments rather than spanning the radiocarpal joint to the index finger metacarpal. The purpose of this article is to review the contemporary use of nonbridging external fixation for the treatment of distal radius fractures.

BRIDGING EXTERNAL FIXATION

No discussion of nonbridging external fixation for the distal radius can be complete without initially discussing radiocarpal bridging external fixation. Bridging external fixation for fractures of the distal radius was first described in 1944.[20] Historically, treatment of distal radius fractures with reduction and casting suffered from an inconsistent ability to maintain satisfactory fracture positioning, particularly in inherently unstable fractures.[21-23] Bridging external fixation grew to become one of the standard methods for treating unstable distal radius injuries.[7,24,25] In this technique, distractive forces across the carpus

The Philadelphia Hand Center, P.C., Thomas Jefferson University Hospital, 834 Chestnut Street, Suite G114, Philadelphia, PA 19107, USA
* Corresponding author.
E-mail address: ekshin@handcenters.com

Hand Clin 26 (2010) 381–390
doi:10.1016/j.hcl.2010.04.006

hand.theclinics.com

achieve and maintain reduction of fracture fragments through ligamentotaxis.[26,27]

This method of indirect reduction relies primarily on tension through the radioscaphocapitate and long radiolunate ligaments.[26] Stress relaxation of these ligaments after radius reduction can occur due to the inherent viscoelastic properties of ligament tissue. Ultimately, this results in diminished distractive forces across the fracture site, potentially causing a loss of satisfactory reduction.[26,28–30] The initial improvements in radial height, radial inclination, and palmar tilt are commonly decreased by the time of fixator removal (**Table 1**).[31] Furthermore, because the volar radiocarpal ligaments are shorter and stouter than the dorsal ligaments, reduction of distal radius fractures by ligamentotaxis is frequently incomplete and fails to adequately correct dorsal angulation of the distal fracture segment.[32–34] Use of bridging external fixation in this scenario is problematic because final functional recovery correlates with restoration of normal carpal alignment.[35–37]

In addition to the difficulties encountered in obtaining and maintaining adequate reduction of distal radius fractures with radiocarpal traction and ligamentotaxis, bridging external fixation is concerning in other areas. Excessive longitudinal traction while attempting reduction can lead to overdistraction after fixator placement (**Fig. 1**). The development of wrist stiffness has been associated with the magnitude and period of distraction.[38] Furthermore, increased carpal tunnel pressures have been measured in the overly distracted wrist, potentially causing acute carpal tunnel syndrome.[39] The elaborate nature of carpal kinematics and the difficulty associated with maintaining adequate ligamentotaxis through the full

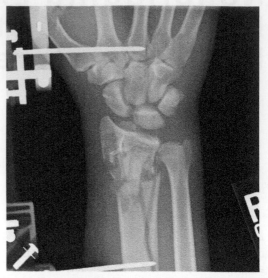

Fig. 1. Excessive longitudinal traction using a bridging external fixation device.

range of motion has contributed to poor success using dynamic bridging external fixation systems for distal radius fractures.[40,41] Consequently, despite contemporary recognition that postreduction carpal function is aided by early motion, bridging external fixation has been largely unable to meet this criteria.

McQueen and colleagues[42] reported on a series of 28 patients with 31 fractures who underwent spanning external fixation as definitive care. Their results revealed a 50% complication rate overall. Patients also exhibited disappointing hand function with regard to grip strength and ability to perform activities of daily living despite radiographically tolerable union positions. There was a close correlation between the complication rate and the incidence of reduced grip strength: statistical significance ($P<.005$) was noted between the complication rate and its effect on patients with weak grip strengths (11/14, 79%) versus those with normal grip strengths (3/17, 18%).

Nonbridging external fixation evolved to provide an external fixation method that reduces these difficulties and improves on the results associated with carpus-spanning fixation. The ability of nonbridging fixation to obtain and maintain reduction of distal radius fractures—including restoration of normal palmar tilt and radial height—is a key contribution to the theoretic successes with this technique.

INDICATIONS/CONTRAINDICATIONS

Nonbridging external fixation is indicated for the treatment of unstable distal radius fractures at

Table 1
Radiographic criteria for acceptable healing of a distal radius fracture

Radiographic Criterion	Acceptable Measurement
Radioulnar length	Radial shortening of <5 mm at distal radioulnar joint compared with contralateral wrist
Radial inclination	Inclination on posteroanterior film >15°
Volar tilt	Sagittal angulation on lateral projection between 15° dorsal tilt and 20° volar tilt
Articular incongruity	Incongruity of intra-articular fracture <2 mm at radiocarpal joint

high risk for late collapse and subsequent mal-union. The work of Lafontaine and colleagues[43] identified several risk factors associated with subsequent instability in the setting of a satisfactory initial reduction. These included patient age greater than 60 years, dorsal fragment angulation greater than 20°, dorsal cortical comminution, radiocarpal articular involvement, and concomitant ulna fracture. Fracture collapse was increasingly likely in the presence of more than 3 of these risk factors. Mackenney and colleagues[5] further reinforced the importance of patient age, dorsal metaphyseal comminution, and ulnar variance in predicting instability and malunion risk (**Table 2**). Ultimately, the identification of notable fracture displacement on injury radiographs predisposes to loss of reduction and fracture malunion even after a successful initial reduction with restoration of normal anatomic relationships.

A distal radius fracture with distal fragments too diminutive for pin placement is a contraindication to the use of nonbridging external fixation. The extensive work of McQueen[37,44] on nonbridging external fixation has suggested that at least 1 cm of intact volar cortex is required for satisfactory pin purchase. The presence of dorsal comminution does not preclude a successful result, although fractures with significant metaphyseal or diaphyseal comminution may require supplemental internal fixation. The use of nonbridging external fixation is also contraindicated in skeletally immature patients with open distal radial physes. Distal radius fractures with volar or volar shear displacement patterns are better treated with alternative reduction and fixation methods.[44]

Recent investigation has examined the success of extending the use of nonbridging external fixation to the treatment of intra-articular distal radius fractures. Nonbridging external fixation permits early joint motion, thereby promoting cartilage reparative processes and diminished wrist stiffness.[45,46] Early motion also helps prevent distal fragment osteopenia.[47] Biomechanical studies reported by Slutsky[26,30] on the characteristics of the Fragment Specific Fixator (South Bay Hand Surgery Center, Torrance, CA, USA) (**Fig. 2**) have confirmed the device's ability to maintain fixation for 2- and 3-part intra-articular distal radius fractures.

AVAILABLE SYSTEMS

Several contemporary systems are available to stabilize distal radius fractures with nonbridging external fixation. The development of nonbridging external fixation as a technique generally predates the existence of dedicated nonbridging systems. Consequently, the initial experience with nonbridging distal radius fixation required standard carpus-bridging fixators to be used to create nonbridging constructs. The Hoffmann II Compact external fixator (Stryker, Kalamazoo, MI, USA) is a modular system that uses threaded pins for purchase into bone. It is indicated for use in the treatment of extra-articular and intra-articular distal radius fractures. Nonbridging fixation is facilitated through the use of 3-mm pins that attach to a proprietary periarticular pin clamp. The radiolucent periarticular pin clamp that is stabilized via connecting rods to a pin and clamp construct proximal to the fracture on the radial diaphysis. The nonspanning wrist frame version of the Small External Fixator (Synthes, Paoli, PA, USA) similarly uses standard bridging external fixator componentry to achieve nonbridging fixation. Bone penetration is achieved with several self-drilling Schanz screws or Kirschner (K) wires. Clamp and connecting rod components complete the construct and provide radioradial external fixation. Bridging or nonbridging external fixation of distal radius fractures can be performed with both of these systems in their usual conformations.

Dedicated systems for providing nonbridging external fixation of distal radius fractures have recently become increasingly available. A cross-pin fixation system (CPX, AM Surgical, Smithtown, NY, USA) is indicated for use in the management of displaced or nondisplaced distal radius fractures with a minimal to moderate degree of comminution. Although fixation into bone is obtained exclusively with 1.6-mm K-wires, the essential component of the CPX is a 2-part sliding aluminum bar with 2 screws to adjust the construct length. Adjustable terminal heads attach at either end, each with 3 adjustable K-wire fixation sites. The K-wire fixators possess 2 screws: one screw

---

Table 2
Radiographic criteria for distal radius fracture instability at presentation

Radiographic Criterion	Value/Type
Comminution	>50% from Dorsal to volar Palmar metaphyseal comminution
Angulation	>20° Dorsal tilt
Shortening	>10 mm
Fracture pattern	Shearing, carpal fracture dislocation (Barton) Intra-articular disruption Associated ulna fracture
Displacement	>100% loss of opposition

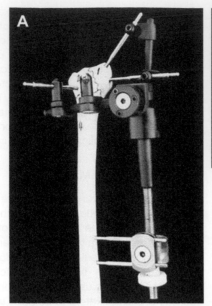
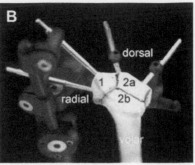

Fig. 2. (*A, B*) Fragment Specific Fixator (South Bay Hand Surgery Center, Torrance, CA, USA) demonstrating pin configuration in an intra-articular fracture. *From* Slutsky DJ. Non-bridging external fixation of intra-articular distal radius fractures. Hand Clin 2005;21:381–94; with permission.

allows adjustment for the angle of wire insertion of up to 10° around a center insertion point; the second permits secure locking of the K-wires to the fixator. Similar to the CPX, the NBX fixator (Nutek Orthopaedics, Fort Lauderdale, FL, USA) relies on 1.6-mm K-wires for purchase into bone at the distal radius fracture site. The NBX body is a radiolucent, dorsally placed polycarbonate device that locks a matrix of dorsally introduced K-wires about the distal radius fracture. An additional outrigger permits the additional placement of K-wires in a radial-to-ulnar direction that interdigitate with the dorsally introduced pins. Radial diaphyseal fixation is obtained with 3-mm threaded pins and distal translation is performed across the fracture site before final tightening with the aid of a threaded distraction device that screws into the polycarbonate plate. The Fragment Specific Fixator is a customizable, nonbridging external fixation device with an integrated dorsal sidearm that uses threaded half-pins to achieve stable fixation of distal radius fractures. Use for extra-articular and intra-articular fractures without severe comminution is indicated. Results documenting the success of several of these systems in achieving and maintaining adequate fixation have been published.[26,27,30]

SURGICAL TECHNIQUE

The technique used for fixation of the fractured distal radius with the NBX is representative of the method used for successful treatment using nonbridging external fixation. After the induction of satisfactory anesthesia and surgical draping, closed reduction of the fracture is performed and confirmed with the assistance of image intensification. The fixation device is positioned over the dorsal wrist and radius, and intraoperative fluoroscopy is again used to confirm appropriate positioning. A series of 1.5-mm dorsal-to-volar fixation pins or K-wires is inserted under fluoroscopic guidance into the radius fracture fragments taking care to avoid penetration of the distal radius articular surface. The first pin is inserted at the most distal ulnar corner of the radius and is followed by a radial styloid fragment pin. Periarticular fracture fragments ideally have fixation pins placed in a juxta-articular position adjacent to the subchondral plate for maximal bony purchase. Bone graft may be necessary to fill any metaphyseal defects. The fixation device is lifted 1 to 2 cm from the skin surface and locked into position on the pins. Depending on the nonbridging fixator system in use, additional pins perpendicular to the dorsal-to-volar pins can be inserted in a radial-to-ulnar direction to provide additional fracture support and stability when locking into the construct.

Fixation on the radial shaft proximal to the fracture site is obtained with an initial 3-mm pin. Gentle distraction is then used to fine-tune the restoration of radial height, radial inclination, and volar tilt initially obtained after closed reduction. A second 3-mm proximal pin is introduced into the radial shaft, and the fixator is locked onto both proximal pins. After final confirmation of ideal fracture reduction with image intensification and locking of all pin attachments to the fixator device, the pins are cut short and the skin insertion sites dressed appropriately (**Fig. 3**).

After surgery, unrestricted wrist motion is allowed. Pin care is emphasized to prevent infection. Oral antibiotics are generally not necessary unless pin tract infection is observed. Assuming appropriate fracture healing radiographically, the fixator may be removed approximately 6 weeks after the index procedure. Physiotherapy may be instituted to maximize upper extremity mobility and strength (**Fig. 4**).

PATIENT OUTCOMES
Nonbridging External Fixation Series

McQueen[37] first introduced the nonbridging concept of external fixation in 1998. She concluded, in her randomized prospective study of 60 patients, that nonbridging external fixation was superior to bridging external fixation regarding anatomic and functional outcomes. Subsequent to her initial report, several case series have evaluated the efficacy of nonbridging external fixation for treatment of extra-articular and intra-articular fractures. These patient series are mostly restricted to the European literature.

Gradl and colleagues[48] reported on 25 consecutive patients with distal radius fractures who were treated with nonbridging external fixation for 6 weeks. Final clinical and radiographic evaluation occurred at 2 years after surgery. At final evaluation, all fractures had united with a palmar tilt greater than 0° and an articular step-off less than 2 mm. Fractures in 4 patients in which only 3 wires were inserted in the distal fragment revealed a loss of radial height. Conversely, radial shortening was not observed in fractures treated with the insertion of 4 wires into the distal fragment. Patients exhibited an average of 55° extension and 64° flexion without appreciable differences between extra-articular and intra-articular fractures. Pin loosening and extensor tendonitis were not noted; however, there were 3 cases of pin tract infections. Gartland and Werley score assessments at 2 years revealed 3 good and 20 excellent results.

A recent study by Andersen and colleagues[49] reviewed the results of nonbridging external fixation in a population of 105 patients with distal radius extra-articular fractures. Despite the loss of 30 patients to follow-up, 75 patients continued for evaluation at 1 year. Independent reviewers using the modified Gartland and Werley system reported good to excellent results in 66 patients (88%). Three patients (4%) required repeat surgery in the initial treatment period for fracture collapse, but all patients maintained satisfactory

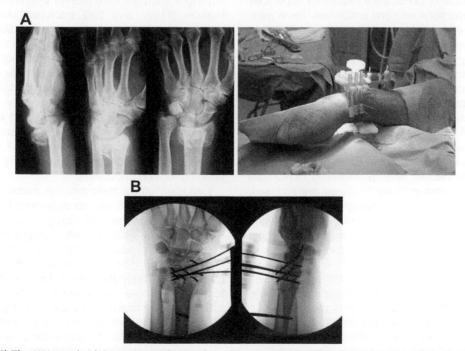

Fig. 3. (*A*) The NBX nonbridging external fixator (Nutek Orthopaedics, Fort Lauderdale, FL, USA) allows fixation of intra-articular distal radius injuries using multiple K-wires, which interlock distally. (*B*) Intraoperative photograph after distal radius stabilization using the NBX fixator. *Courtesy of* Mohamad A. Hajianpour, MD.

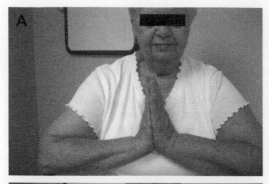

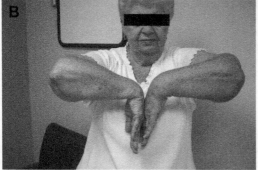

Fig. 4. (*A*, *B*) Postoperative clinical photographs demonstrating final motion after nonbridging fixator removal. *Courtesy of* Mohamad A. Hajianpour, MD.

radiographic criteria for radial length, angulation, and inclination at interval and final follow-up. Twenty patients (31%) were treated for superficial pin site infections with oral antibiotics. There were no deep infections requiring pin removal. Carpal tunnel syndrome and reflex sympathetic dystrophy were not reported in the study population, although extensor pollicis longus tendon rupture occurred during the follow-up period.

Mirza and colleagues[27] reported their experiences using the CPX system, a nonbridging external fixation device that stabilizes and locks percutaneously using crossing K-wires distally. Twenty-one distal radius fractures spanning a range of fracture severity, including 15 AO type C complex intra-articular fractures, were closed, reduced, and stabilized. Longitudinal evaluation of radiographic parameters, including radial height, palmar tilt, radial inclination, and ulnar variance, demonstrated no loss of reduction at final follow-up. Active range of motion recovered to at least 89% of the uninjured side. Additionally, patient mean grip and pinch strength returned to 86% and 94% of the contralateral limb, respectively.

Surveys of patient functional recovery and satisfaction (disabilities of the arm, shoulder and hand [DASH] and patient-rated wrist evaluation [PRWHE]) demonstrated resumption of usual activities and return of functional status early in the recovery period. No pin tract infections, loss of reduction, or tendon ruptures were reported. Recorded complications included radial sensory neuritits and chronic regional pain syndrome, which resolved with conservative management. One case of late carpal tunnel syndrome in a multiply injured patient was also identified and ultimately required endoscopic carpal tunnel release and wrist manipulation. The investigators concluded that the CPX system is a minimally invasive technique that allows for stable fixation of distal radius injuries, early wrist immobilization, and predictable outcomes. They also emphasized the manageable learning curve for the CPX system given most hand surgeons' familiarity with percutaneous pinning techniques.[27]

Comparative External Fixation Series

Patient series comparing the efficacy of bridging versus nonbridging external fixation are spare and conflicting. Hayes and colleagues[50] reported on their experiences with 588 patients who underwent bridging and nonbridging external fixation in the treatment of unstable distal radius fractures. The investigators attempted nonbridging external fixation for the treatment of primary and secondary fracture instability unless the operating surgeon felt that the distal fragment was insufficiently large to accomodate pin placement. Three hundred fifty-eight fractures were treated with nonbridging fixation (61%), and 230 fractures underwent bridging fixation. Analysis of the radiographic results revealed that fractures treated with bridging fixation were significantly more likely than those treated with nonbridging fixation to undergo dorsal malunion and unsatisfactory radial shortening (*P*<.001). The odds ratio after adjustment for confounding factors revealed a 6-fold increased malunion risk in the bridging versus nonbridging fixation group. Similarly, the risk of radial shortening was 2.5 times more likely in the bridging fixation population.

Excluding dorsal malunion, the overall complication rate was 22% with minor pin tract infections more common in the nonbridging group (*P*<.001). Ruptures of the extensor pollicis longus occurred in 1% of the fractures treated in both groups. There were no differences between the 2 treatment groups regarding the incidence of carpal tunnel syndrome or chronic regional pain syndrome. The investigators concluded that nonbridging fixation reduces the risk of dorsal malunion compared with bridging external fixation.[50]

Hayes and colleagues study represents the largest series of patients comparing bridging versus nonbridging external fixation. Other comparative studies, however, have been unable to confirm their findings and do not definitively illustrate the superiority of nonbridging fixation.

In a prospective, randomized study of 60 patients, Krishnan and colleagues[51] compared bridging fixation with the Hoffmann II Compact external fixator to nonbridging fixation provided by the AO Delta frame (Synthes, Paoli, PA, USA). Results between the 2 groups were similar with no statistically significant differences at any stage in evaluations of extension, ulnar deviation, forearm supination, and forearm pronation. The nonbridging group demonstrated significantly increased radial deviation at 6 weeks postoperatively ($P = .002$), whereas the Hoffmann bridging group showed significantly more wrist flexion at 6 weeks ($P = .02$), 26 weeks ($P = .008$), and 52 weeks ($P = .02$). Complication rates between the groups were similar with pin site infection occurring most commonly (19 patients, 32%). In conclusion, this study demonstrated that the outcomes of patients with complex unstable intra-articular fractures of the distal radius are similar, regardless of whether or not they are treated with a static bridging external fixator or a dynamic nonbridging external fixator.

A prospective, randomized study by Atroshi and colleagues[52] compared the treatment of extra-articular and minimally comminuted intra-articular distal radius fractures with bridging and nonbridging external fixation. Using DASH scores as the primary investigative endpoint in a population of women aged over 50 years and men aged over 60 years, the investigators found no significant difference between the 2 study groups, totaling 38 patients. Secondary outcomes were also evaluated and included wrist range of motion, grip strength, pain, and overall patient satisfaction. No statistically significant differences were found between the 2 groups at 52 weeks' follow-up. A statistically insignificant incidence of superficial pin site infections amenable to treatment with oral antibiotics was the most frequently encountered complication in both groups. There were no cases of carpal tunnel syndrome, complex regional pain syndrome, or tendon ruptures.

Finally, a 2009 Norwegian study randomized 75 patients to nonbridging external fixation with the Hoffmann II fixator or the dynamic bridging Dynawrist fixator (Prototech AS, Bergen, Norway) for the surgical management of unstable distal radius fractures. Evaluation of radiographic criteria, wrist range of motion, return of function as assessed by DASH score and visual analog scale (VAS)-quantified pain was assessed. Review of radiographs postoperatively and at fixator removal revealed the nonbridging construct better recreated the radial volar tilt than the dynamic fixator ($P = .002$ and $P = .04$, respectively). The differences between the 2 systems were not statistically significant by final follow-up at 1 year. Evaluation of ulnar variance and radial inclination failed to identify statistically significant differences between the 2 groups. Although wrist flexion was better at 6 weeks in the dynamic fixator group, the difference was insignificant at subsequent review out to 1 year. Final follow-up at 52 weeks also revealed no statistically significant differences between the VAS and DASH scores. Complications were limited to superficial pin site infections and transient superficial radial nerve injury in both treatment groups.[53]

Fracture Malunion

A 2008 study by McQueen and Wakefield[54] took successful use of nonbridging fixation for distal radius fractures and applied it to fixation of osteotomies for treatment of malunions. The investigators report on radiographic, functional, and patient-assessed outcomes at 6 months after distal radial osteotomy using nonbridging external fixation and bone grafting for dorsally malunited, extra-articular distal radius fractures. The study group comprised 23 patients with a median age of 60 (18–84) years. A correction from a mean preoperative dorsal angle of 20° (5°–40°) to greater than 5° (0°–15°) of volar tilt ($P<.001$) was obtained. Mean preoperative positive ulnar variance of 3.9 (0–8) mm was corrected to 2.5 (0–8) mm ($P = .005$). Twenty-two of the 23 patients ultimately had correction of their carpal alignment. Simultaneous ulna surgery was required for 5 patients: 1 required ulnar shortening and 4 required modified Bowers procedures. All measures of function except extension and key grip strength showed statistically significant improvements in their means by 6 months postoperatively. Short form 36 scores showed statistical improvements in 2 domains, role physical and bodily pain. Two patients experienced extensor pollicis longus ruptures, and 13 developed minor pin tract infections.

SUMMARY

Distal radius injuries are the most common fracture of the upper extremity in adults. The management of these injuries has evolved as more information about patient outcomes becomes available. An increase in the size of the elderly population and an increasingly active elderly population portends an escalation in the number of osteoporotic distal radius fractures. A recent trend has seen the increasing use of volar internal fixation for the treatment of distal radius fractures.

External fixation, however, continues to have a treatment role in the contemporary management of distal radius fractures. Nonbridging fixation represents the most recent external fixation development for anatomic fracture reduction and early initiation of range-of-motion physiotherapy.

Standard bridging external fixation for distal radius fractures has been used since its initial description in 1944. Ligamentotaxis across the carpus is used to obtain and maintain reduction of the fracture with this method. Inherent viscoelastic properties of ligament tissue and shorter, thicker volar carpal ligaments contribute to the common inability of bridging external fixation to maintain satisfactory radial height and volar tilt. Additional complications associated with the use of standard bridging radiocarpal fixation include excessive traction and wrist stiffness.

Nonbridging external fixation is indicated for the treatment of unstable distal radius fractures at high risk for late collapse and subsequent malunion. Nonbridging fixation is contraindicated in skeletally immature patients with open distal radial physes. Although originally developed for use in extra-articular fractures, new products and procedures have extended nonbridging external fixation to the management of intra-articular injuries, too. The surgical technique for nonbridging fixation relies on successful placement of pins into individual fracture fragments and closed reduction to restore radial height and volar tilt. Nonbridging fixation allows early mobilization of the forearm, wrist, and fingers while maintaining anatomic stability of all fracture fragments.

Despite its theoretic advantages, nonbridging fixation has some limitations: at least 1 cm of intact volar cortex is required for satisfactory pin purchase, the operative technique is more demanding, and there is a risk of damaging the extensor tendons. There is also possibly an increased risk of infection in the tendon sheaths, the fracture zone, or the wrist joint as compared with bridging fixators. Finally, nonbridging fixation has not been shown definitively to improve patient outcomes relative to traditional spanning external fixators. Although early motion may be improved with nonbridging constructs, comparative studies featuring long-term follow-up demonstrated no significant differences in wrist mobility and with patient-measured outcomes.

REFERENCES

1. Owen RA, Melton LJ, Johnson KA, et al. Incidence of Colles' fracture in a North American community. Am J Public Health 1982;72(6):605–7.

2. Chung KC, Spilson SV. The frequency and epidemiology of hand and forearm fractures in the United States. J Hand Surg Am 2001;26:908–15.

3. Colles A. On the fracture of the carpal extremity of the radius. Edinburgh Med Surg J 1814;10:182.

4. Beharrie AW, Beredjiklian PK, Bozentka DJ. Functional outcomes after open reduction and internal fixation for treatment of displaced distal radius fractures in patients over 60 years of age. J Orthop Trauma 2004;18:680–6.

5. Mackenney PJ, McQueen MM, Elton R. Prediction of instability in distal radial fractures. J Bone Joint Surg Am 2006;88:1944–51.

6. Strange-Vognsen HH. Intraarticular fractures of the distal end of the radius in young adults. A 16 (2–26) year follow-up of 42 patients. Acta Orthop Scand 1991;62:527–30.

7. Chung KC, Shauver MJ, Birkmeyer JD. Trends in the United States in the treatment of distal radial fractures in the elderly. J Bone Joint Surg Am 2009;91: 1868–73.

8. Bradway JK, Amadio PC, Cooney WP. Open reduction and internal fixation of displaced, comminuted intra-articular fractures of the distal end of the radius. J Bone Joint Surg Am 1989; 71:839–47.

9. Fernandez DL, Jupiter JB. Epidemiology, mechanism, classification. In: Fernandez DL, Jupiter JB, editors. Fractures of the distal radius: a practical approach to management. New York: Springer-Verlag; 2002. p. 24–5.

10. Itoh S, Tomioka H, Tanaka J, et al. Relationship between bone mineral density of the distal radius and ulna and fracture characteristics. J Hand Surg Am 2004;29:123–30.

11. Jakob M, Rikli DA, Regazzoni P. Fractures of the distal radius treated by internal fixation and early function, a prospective study of 73 consecutive patients. J Bone Joint Surg Br 2000;82:340–4.

12. Kambouroglou GK, Axelrod TS. Complications of the AO/ASIF titanium distal radius plate system (Pi plate) in internal fixation of the distal radius: a brief report. J Hand Surg Am 1998;23:737–41.

13. Orbay J, Badia A, Khoury RK, et al. Volar fixed-angle fixation of distal radius fractures: the DVR plate. Tech Hand Up Extrem Surg 2004;8:142–8.

14. Jupiter JB. Commentary on "Improvement of the bone-pin interface strength in osteoporotic bone with hydroxyapatite-coated tapered external fixation pins by Antonio Moroni, MD et al J Bone Joint Surg Am 83 5 [about 1p]. Available at: http://www.jbjs. org/Comments/c_p_jupiter.shtml. Accessed October 23, 2009.

15. Cummings SR, Black DM, Rubin SM. Lifetime risks of hip, Colles', or vertebral fracture and coronary heart disease among white postmenopausal women. Arch Intern Med 1989;149:2445–8.

16. Drobetz H, Kutscha-Lissberg E. Osteosynthesis of distal radius fractures with a volar locking scew plate system. Int Orthop 2003;27:1–6.

17. Koval KJ, Harrast JJ, Anglen JO, et al. Fractures of the distal part of the radius. The evolution of practice over time. Where's the evidence? J Bone Joint Surg Am 2008;90:1855–61.

18. Orbay JL. The treatment of unstable distal radius fractures with volar fixation. Hand Surg 2000;5: 103–12.

19. Slutsky DJ. A comparison of external vs. internal fixation of distal radius fractures. Presented at the American Association of Hand Surgery Annual Meeting. Boca Raton (FL), January 10, 1997.

20. Anderson R, O'Neil G. Comminuted fractures of the distal end of the radius. Surg Gynecol Obstet 1944; 78:434–40.

21. Bindra RR. Biomechanics and biology of external fixation of distal radius fractures. Hand Clin 2005; 21:362–73.

22. Gutow AP. Avoidance of complications of distal radius fractures. Hand Clin 2005;21:295–305.

23. Hanel DP, Jones MD, Trumble TE. Wrist fractures. Orthop Clin North Am 2002;33:35–57.

24. Grana WA, Kopta JA. The Roger Anderson device in the treatment of fractures of the distal end of the radius. J Bone Joint Surg Am 1979;61:1234–8.

25. Vaughan PA, Lui SM, Harrington IJ, et al. Treatment of unstable fractures of the distal radius by external fixation. J Bone Joint Surg Br 1985;67:385–9.

26. Slutsky DJ. External fixation of distal radius fractures. J Hand Surg Am 2007;32:1624–37.

27. Mirza A, Jupiter JB, Reinhart MK, et al. Fractures of the distal radius treated with cross pin fixation and a non-bridging external fixator, the CPX system: a preliminary report. J Hand Surg Am 2009;34:603–16.

28. Winemaker MJ, Chinchalkar S, Richards RS, et al. Load relaxation and forces with activity in Hoffman external fixators: a clinical study in patients with Colles' fractures. J Hand Surg Am 1998;23:926–32.

29. Woo SL, Gomez MA, Akeson WH. The time and history-dependent viscoelastic properties of the canine medial collateral ligament. J Biomech Eng 1981;103:293–8.

30. Slutsky DJ. Non-bridging external fixation of intra-articular distal radius fractures. Hand Clin 2005;21: 381–94.

31. Sun JS, Chang CH, Wu CC, et al. Extra-articular deformity in distal radial fractures treated by external fixation. Can J Surg 2001;44:289–94.

32. Bartosh RA, Saldana MJ. Intraarticular fractures of the distal radius: a cadaveric study to determine if ligamentoataxis restores radiopalmar tilt. J Hand Surg Am 1990;15:18–21.

33. Fernandez DL, Geissler WB. Treatment of displaced articular fractures of the radius. J Hand Surg Am 1991;16:375–84.

34. Sanders RA, Keppel FL, Waldrop JI. External fixation of distal radial fractures: results and complications. J Hand Surg Am 1991;16:385–91.

35. Taleisnik J, Watson HK. Midcarpal instability caused by malunited fractures of the distal radius. J Hand Surg Am 1984;9:350–7.

36. McQueen MM, Hajducka C, Court-Brown CM. Re-displaced unstable fractures of the distal radius: a prospective randomised comparison of four methods of treatment. J Bone Joint Surg Br 1996; 78:404–9.

37. McQueen MM. Redisplaced unstable fractures of the distal radius: a randomised, prospective study of bridging versus non-bridging external fixation. J Bone Joint Surg Br 1998;80:665–9.

38. Kaempffe FA, Wheeler DR, Palmer CA, et al. Severe fractures of the distal radius: effect of amount and duration of external fixator distraction on outcome. J Hand Surg Am 1993;18:33–41.

39. Baechler MF, Means KR Jr, Parks BG, et al. Carpal canal pressure of the distracted wrist. J Hand Surg Am 2004;29:858–64.

40. Sommerkamp TG, Seeman M, Sillman J, et al. Dynamic external fixation of unstable fractures of the the the distal part of the radius. A prospective, randomized comparison with static external fixation. J Bone Joint Surg Am 1994;76:1149–61.

41. Kawaguchi S, Sawada K, Nabeta Y, et al. Recurrent dorsal angulation of the distal radius fracture during dynamic external fixation. J Hand Surg Am 1998;23: 920–5.

42. McQueen MM, Michie M, Court-Brown CM. Hand and wrist function after external fixation of unstable distal radial fractures. Clin Orthop Relat Res 1992; 285:200–4.

43. Lafontaine M, Hardy D, Delince P. Stability assessment of distal radial fractures. Injury 1989;208: 208–10.

44. McQueen MM. Non-spanning external fixation of the distal radius. Hand Clin 2005;21:375–80.

45. Salter RB, Simmonds DF, Malcolm BW, et al. The biological effect of continuous passive motion on the healing of full-thickness defects in articular carti-lage. An experimental investigation in the rabbit. J Bone Joint Surg Am 1980;62:1232–51.

46. Salter RB. The physiologic effects of continuous passive motion for articular cartilage healing and regeneration. Hand Clin 1994;10:211–9.

47. Mehta JA, Slavotinek JP, Krishnan J. Local osteoppenia associated with the management of intra-articular distal radial fractures by insertion of external fixation pins in the distal fragment: a prospective study. J Orthop Surg (Hong Kong) 2002;10:179–84.

48. Gradl G, Jupiter JB, Gierer P. Fractures of the distal radius treated with a non-bridging external fixation technique using mulitplanar K-wires. J Hand Surg Am 2005;30:960–8.

49. Andersen JK, Hogh A, Gantov J, et al. Colles fracture treated with non-bridging external fixation: a 1 year follow-up. J Hand Surg Br 2009;34:475–8.

50. Hayes AJ, Duffy PJ, McQueen MM. Bridging and non-bridging external fixation in the treatment of unstable fractures of the distal radius: A retrospective study of 588 patients. Acta Orthop 2008;79: 540–7.

51. Krishnan J, Wigg AER, Walker RW, et al. Intra-articular fractures of the distal radius: a prospective randomised controlled trial comparing static bridging and non-bridging external fixation. J Hand Surg Br 2003;28:417–21.

52. Atroshi I, Brogren E, Larsson GU, et al. Wrist-bridging versus non-bridging external fixation for displaced distal radius fractures: A randomized assessor-blind clinical trial of 38 patients followed for 1 year. Acta Orthop 2006;77:445–53.

53. Krukhaug Y, Ugland S, Lie SA, et al. External fixation of fractures of the distal radius: A randomized comparison of the Hoffman compact II non-bridging fixator and the Dynawrist fixator in 75 patients followed for 1 year. Acta Orthop 2009;80:104–8.

54. McQueen MM, Wakefield A. Distal radial osteotomy for malunion using non-bridging external fixation: Good results in 23 patients. Acta Orthop 2008;79:390–5.

Intramedullary Fixation of Forearm Fractures

Saqib Rehman, MD[a,b,*], Gbolabo Sokunbi, MD[a]

KEYWORDS

• Forearm fracture • Intramedullary nailing • Radius • Ulna

Treatment options for forearm fractures include closed management and various surgical treatment methods. Fracture pattern, patient age, soft-tissue envelope integrity, and other factors help guide the surgeon's decision on how to treat these common injuries. Nevertheless, the goal of treatment is to maintain length and radioulnar joint relationships to regain full pronosupination. In the adult, combined radius and ulna both-bones forearm fractures are usually treated with operative fixation to achieve these goals. Nonoperative management of these injuries is typically reserved for the pediatric population and the uncommon nondisplaced fracture pattern. It has long been recognized that nonoperative management of forearm fractures in adults typically leads to unacceptable outcomes. Even in minimally displaced fractures, the deforming forces typically lead to shortening and angulation.[1] Bagley reported poor results with closed management of forearm fractures in 1928.[2] Similar results with closed management were still being reported in the 1950s by Bolton and Hughston in 2 separate reports.[3,4] In 1945, Evans had somewhat acceptable results with plaster immobilization, but even 30% of their patients lost at least 50° of pronosupination.[5] It has now been long recognized that these poor outcomes are directly related to loss of anatomic length and radial bow. Deformity of

the radius or ulna can directly result in impaired rotational mechanics at the proximal and distal radioulnar joints. As a result, anatomic reduction of these diaphyseal fractures has been emphasized to maintain these important anatomic relationships.

Compression plate techniques as advocated by the arbeitsgemeinschaft für osteosynthesefragen/association for the study of internal fixation (AO/ASIF) group have become the surgical treatment of choice in simple adult forearm fracture patterns. Bridge plating methods have also been used in more complex fracture patterns. Although intramedullary (IM) nailing has become commonplace in lower extremity diaphyseal fractures and is performed with regularity in humeral shaft fractures, the forearm remains the only major diaphyseal segment in which this technique is seldom employed.

Early nailing techniques included various nonlocked implants, such as Rush rods and Kirschner wires. These methods have been associated with nonunion rates up to 21% likely caused by the lack of rotational and axial stability, the latter being more problematic in comminuted fractures.[6] More recently, implants designed specifically for intramedullary nailing have had more success. The authors hereby describe the history, indications, surgical techniques, and results of treatment of forearm

No funding or support has been provided for this study.
a Department of Orthopaedic Surgery, Temple University Hospital, 6th Floor, Outpatient Building, 3401 North Broad Street, Philadelphia, PA 19140, USA
b Department of Anatomy and Cell Biology, Temple University School of Medicine, 3500 North Broad Street, Philadelphia, PA 19140, USA
* Corresponding author. Department of Orthopaedic Surgery, Temple University Hospital, 6th Floor, Outpatient Building, 3401 North Broad Street, Philadelphia, PA 19140.
E-mail address: saqib.rehman@tuhs.temple.edu

Hand Clin 26 (2010) 391–401
doi:10.1016/j.hcl.2010.04.002

fractures by intramedullary nailing methods. Although flexible nailing procedures in children and adolescents is a common technique for certain indications, this is not discussed in this article.

HISTORY AND RESULTS WITH UNLOCKED NAILING

The anatomy of the forearm is part of the reason that intramedullary nailing has been historically problematic. Restoration of function, mainly the reestablishment of pronosupination, is highly dependent on the restoration of length, rotational alignment, and anatomic bow of the radius. The interdependence of 2 bones (the radius and ulna) and the bow of the radius have made intramedullary fixation difficult. Straight implants can work well in the ulna because of its slightly S-shaped but straight morphology. However, placing straight implants, such as simple Kirchner wires and Rush rods, in the radius can effectively eliminate the anatomic bow, which can result in malunion and loss of pronosupination of the forearm.

Open reduction and internal fixation (ORIF) with plate fixation has been the recommended treatment for these injuries by the AO/ASIF group. In fact, management of these diaphyseal fractures has been considered analogous to that of articular fractures in that anatomic reduction is required to restore function. Furthermore, plates do not need to be anatomically shaped and they facilitate compression. ORIF of these injuries is a reliable procedure with more than acceptable union rates with few complications. In 1975, Anderson and colleagues[7] reported on 244 subjects with forearm fractures treated with AO compression plates with 98% union rate of the radius and 96% union rate of the ulna. Similarly, Chapman and colleagues[8] reported on 129 forearm fractures treated with 3.5-mm AO dynamic compression plates with 98% union rate and 92% satisfactory or excellent results. In both cases, autogenous bone grafting was used acutely when necessary. As demonstrated in both of these studies, compression plating has justifiably become the treatment of choice in most diaphyseal forearm fractures. However, intramedullary nailing was done before 3.5-mm AO plating in North America.

Intramedullary nailing in the forearm has been reported as early as 1913 with unsatisfactory results.[9] Rush and Rush reported on the use of intramedullary pinning in the proximal ulna in 1937.[10] Their pins were modified over time to accommodate extended indications for these devices. One of the earlier reports on the use of intramedullary fixation of diaphyseal forearm fractures in North America was in 1952 by Hall and colleagues.[11]

Twenty subjects were treated with supramalleolar orthosis stainless steel pins for ulnar and radius fractures with satisfactory results.

Smith and Sage reported on intramedullary fixation of forearm fractures in 1957.[6] At this time, the AO had still not yet been established and compression plate fixation was not commonplace in North America. However, there had been experience with intramedullary nailing of femoral shaft fractures that spawned interest in similar fixation of forearm fractures. Smith and Sage's report describes results in 338 subjects with 555 forearm fractures from 18 orthopedic centers throughout the United States. All of the surgeons involved were thoroughly acquainted with femoral intramedullary nailing techniques. Multiple techniques were employed: Rush pins, Kirschner wires, Steinmann pins, Kuntscher V nails, and Lottes nails. Problems were noted to be caused by the inability to restore the bowed anatomy of the radius. Only isolated fractures of the ulna had appreciable excellent results (40%). The nonunion rate for all forearm fractures was 21%, with the highest rate in the subgroup including Kirschner-wire fixation (38%). They noted that straightening of the radius led to subsequent lengthening of the ulna and nonunion of both bones (**Fig. 1**). Problems were noted with nonunion and malunion. It was noted that intramedullary fixation, however, provided a good treatment option for the mangled extremity. They concluded that intramedullary fixation was a better option than either plate and screw treatment or other conservative measures because of its ability to maintain length and alignment in these cases.

Sage reported again in 1959 on 50 radius fractures treated with a prebent triangular interference nail.[12] In this series, the overall primary union rate

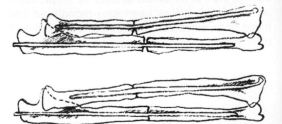

Fig. 1. Insertion of a straight nail into the fractured radius can result in nonanatomic straightening of the radius and subsequent distraction of the ulna as shown in the upper figure. This distraction is a risk factor for nonunion of the ulna. A bowed radial implant maintains radial bow and prevents ulnar distraction as shown in the lower figure. (*Adapted from* Smith H, Sage FP. Medullary fixation of forearm fractures. J Bone Joint Surg 1957;39-A(1):91; with permission.)

(<6 months) was 89%, a significant improvement from that seen with Kirschner wires and other implants as described in their earlier study. Malunion incidence was also reduced in this study, possibly because of the improvements in the implant itself and clinical experience and better understanding of this technique. These prebent nails were an improvement from the straight implants used in other series. To accomplish this, a thorough understanding of the medullary canal was achieved via a cadaveric study sectioning and analyzing one hundred radii reported in this same manuscript. This study highlighted the need for contouring the nails to safely pass the device while accommodating the natural anatomy of the bones. Also highlighted was the importance of the nail design and material constituents. The Ritchey nail was a similar triangular nail used in the forearm with some success.[13] This nail also resembled the Rush pin because of its hook.

In 1954, Street introduced the concept of the interference fit nail that used an oversized nail in a reamed medullary canal.[14] This nail was square-shaped, which was thought to have better rotational control than rounded nails, such as Kirschner wires and Steinman pins. A 7% nonunion rate was reported in this series of 137 nailed fractures in 1986. Closed nailing was the preferred method using the Street square nail.

Rush pinning continued to be practiced during this time period, however. Aho and colleagues[15] reported on 88 forearm fractures in 48 subjects treated with Rush-pin intramedullary nailing from 1966 through 1977. An average of 7.6 years of follow-up was provided with good clinical results in 78% of cases. Delayed union was noted in 5 cases and there were no cases of nonunion. Furthermore, there were no cases of wound infection although comminuted radius fractures did demonstrate shortening.

A union rate of 94% was noted in a series of 70 diaphyseal forearm fractures treated with intramedullary Rush pinning reported in a separate series in 1996 by Moerman and colleagues.[16] This series included fractures of both bones and cases of isolated radius or ulna fractures.

Other methods of using unlocked nails include the Hackethal bundle nailing method of jamming multiple short nails into the medullary cavity. Winckler reported on 65 subjects with 115 forearm fractures treated with this method.[17] There were 71.5% good and excellent, 11.4% satisfactory, and 17.1% poor results with 2.1% infection, 3.1% nonunion, and 2.1% synostosis rates.

In summary, IM nailing has evolved from smooth pinning and Kuntscher techniques with most changes in nail design made to address deficiencies in rotational stability. Union rates and function are generally satisfactory, but most earlier studies have not yielded the consistent success of AO plating techniques. More recent developments with interlocking nailing are discussed later in this article.

BIOMECHANICS

Intramedullary fixation of forearm fractures has been evaluated biomechanically compared with closed treatments and with plate fixation. Rush pinning would not be expected to have significant rotational control of forearm fractures because of their lack of interlocking fixation. However, Rush pinning was found to be at least superior to functional bracing with regard to rotational stability. Ono and colleagues[18] evaluated rotational stability of 6 cadaveric fractured forearms with Rush pinning alone, fracture bracing, fracture bracing with Rush pinning, and with no fixation. Fracture bracing alone provided some rotational stability within specific torque levels. Rush-pin fixation reduced rotational motion to about one eighth of that with no bracing or fixation. The further addition of the brace did not add any further rotational stability.

Limited contact dynamic compression plate fixation was compared biomechanically with fluted intramedullary nails in 8 matched pairs of cadaveric forearms by Jones and colleagues.[19] Medial bending, supination, pronation, axial compression, and distraction loading were performed on all specimens with a materials testing system. They found that the intact ulna contributes more to forearm stability in bending and torsion than does the radius. Therefore, IM nailing of the radius with the intact ulna had greater stiffness, particularly in torsion, than IM nailing of the ulna with the intact radius. If both bones were fractured and fixed with nails, there was significantly less stiffness in torsion (2.23% of intact specimens) compared with plate fixation (83.4% of intact specimens).

INDICATIONS/ADVANTAGES OVER PLATE OSTEOSYNTHESIS

Intramedullary nailing techniques have been performed with success in the adolescent and pediatric population. Most of the experience in this population involves the use of unlocked flexible nails, which can provide adjunctive treatment in patients who would otherwise be treated with casting. In cases in which reduction would be unacceptable with casting alone, or in cases in which earlier range of motion may be desired, flexible unlocked intramedullary nailing can be performed.

In the adult population, plate fixation is generally the preferred technique for treating diaphyseal forearm fractures. Plate fixation of forearm fractures has proven to be successful in achieving adequate reduction and satisfactory healing. There is a large body of literature and years of clinical experience validating its widespread use. Criticism surrounding plate osteosynthesis includes the potential for blood supply disruption and possible inhibition of periosteal revascularization. However, clinical experience with plating has not borne out these fears except in special circumstances. Refracture after plate removal is also a legitimate concern with plate fixation of forearm fractures.

The status of surrounding soft tissues may preclude exposures required for plate fixation. Mangled extremities or burns are situations when traditional open surgical exposures and plate fixation may not be ideal because of the risk for wound complications or deep infection (**Fig. 2**). As recognized more than 50 years ago by Sage and Smith, IM nailing can be a viable option in these cases because of the minimal soft-tissue stripping required for insertion. Analogous to principles applied to the lower extremity, IM nailing spares the periosteal blood supply. Furthermore, the surgical approach is more often remote from the area of soft-tissue injury with lower profile of the implant as opposed to plating techniques (**Fig. 3**).

Segmental diaphyseal fractures are another indication to consider intramedullary nailing. In these cases, plate fixation can often be performed, but might require extensile approaches that may

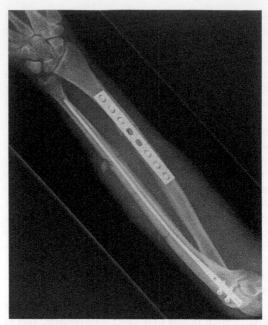

Fig. 3. Intramedullary nailing has been performed in the ulna after initial external fixation and fasciotomies were performed for closed forearm fractures with compartment syndrome. The wound locations did not permit satisfactory access to the ulna for plate fixation without incurring significant additional soft-tissue stripping. Rather than making a third parallel incision with risk of flap necrosis, intramedullary nailing was performed.

not be desirable in certain instances (**Fig. 4**). An intramedullary nail typically is longer than most plates that are used in the forearm. Therefore, although implant length can be a problem when plating segmental fractures, this is not the case when using intramedullary nails.

Pathologic fractures can also be an indication for intramedullary nailing of forearm fractures. In these cases, extensive tumor involvement can require the implant to span the length of the diaphysis. As is the case with pathologic fractures in the diaphysis of other long bones, intramedullary nailing can provide such stability over the length of the bone. In fact, this has been reported in pathologic fractures of the forearm.[20]

Another potential advantage of intramedullary nailing over plating includes the absence of multiple screw holes in the diaphysis, which is a known risk for refracture after forearm plate removal.[21,22] Because of the biomechanical inferiority of most intramedullary nailing methods compared with plate fixation, there is often a need to protect fixation with immobilization for 2 to 4 weeks until radiographic callus formation is evident. This immobilization is a disadvantage when compared with the

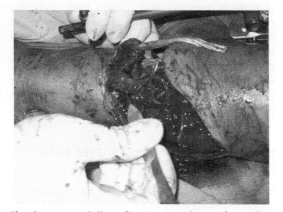

Fig. 2. Intramedullary fixation can be performed in mangled extremities and severe soft-tissue injury. A case of an industrial crush injury with diaphyseal forearm fractures and extensive soft-tissue injury treated with provisional external fixation and serial debridement procedures. Forearm plating in this case would lead to additional unnecessary soft-tissue stripping and would potentially have an increased risk for infection and exposed hardware.

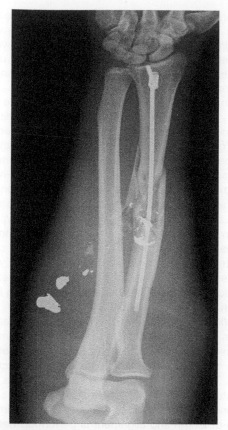

Fig. 4. Intramedullary nailing has been performed in the radius for a segmentally comminuted radial shaft fracture from a low-velocity gunshot injury. A longer nail for improved stability would have been more ideal; however, in this case the intact ulna helps provide some inherent stability.

ability to immediately mobilize patients treated with plate osteosynthesis.

Just as intramedullary fixation can be used in the treatment of deformities in the lower extremity, this can also be done for forearm malunions and nonunions. Although the authors do not advocate this as a routine method for these conditions in the forearm, there are reports of this technique as early as 1976. Kuntscher nailing using a cloverleaf design was used in 20 cases of nonunion of the forearm, with healing in 15 cases.[23] Straight nails were used in this series, including the radius. Infected and aseptic nonunions were treated with this method in this series. In a separate cohort of 30 subjects in 2009 with either pseudarthrosis or refracture of the forearm, intramedullary nailing was done at an average time of 15 months from injury to surgery.[24] Pseudarthrosis was present in 21 subjects and forearm refractures was the problem in the other 9 subjects. Radiographic healing was seen in all subjects at an average of

18.45 weeks after surgery using the Foresight (Smith & Nephew, Memphis, TN, USA) interlocking intramedullary nail system.

Finally, nonunion repair of 15 subjects with 26 nonunions of diaphyseal forearm fractures were treated with the Foresight nailing system and iliac crest bone grafts.[25] Radiographic union was noted in 96% of cases. However, mean loss of wrist flexion and extension was 27° and loss of forearm rotation was 39°. There were only 13% excellent results, with 40% satisfactory results, 40% unsatisfactory results, and 7% failed results. With these results and a mean disabilities of the arm, shoulder, and hand (DASH) score of 35, these investigators did not recommend nailing of nonunions of the forearm despite the favorable union rate.

CONTRAINDICATIONS

As with most internal fixation methods, active infection is a contraindication to intramedullary nailing. As with most intramedullary nailing techniques done elsewhere, canal diameter can also be a limiting factor. Canal diameter smaller than 3 mm is typically a contraindication for intramedullary nailing, although this differs based on the type of implant used.

Open physis in the pediatric/adolescent population precludes the use of large implants that potentially violate these areas. Nails that are intended for immature skeletal fixation should be inserted with portals that spare the physis.

Fracture extension to the metaphysis or articular surface is also a contraindication, particularly if displaced and requiring reduction. Conventional open reduction and internal fixation methods (ie, plate and screw) are indicated in these injuries.

NAIL DESIGN

Forearm nail design has attempted to address the problems previously outlined, including restoring anatomic bow of the radius and allowing interlocking to prevent shortening and rotation. Nails, regardless of the metal used, must possess a modulus of elasticity favoring stiffness for rigidity while being malleable to a degree that ensures safe passage within the medullary canal. McLaren and colleagues[26] recommended that the lower modulus of elasticity of titanium forearm nails facilitates insertion and also provides more load sharing with the bone itself.

The metaphyseal-diaphyseal junction poses an issue for rotational control with the use of interference fit nails. The introduction of static locking has proven a significant advance in the control of unstable rotary forces in the treatment of forearm fractures.

The Foresight nail is a stainless steel nail with a contouring straight shape that has interlocking capability both proximally and distally. These nails are routinely available in 4.0-mm and 5.0-mm diameters. The radius and ulna nails by Acumed (Acumed, Hillsboro, OR, USA) are titanium, precontoured, available in 3.0 and 3.6 mm, and have interlocking capability at the end of insertion (ie, proximally in the ulna, distally in the radius). The True-Flex nail (DJO, Austin, TX, USA) is a titanium prebent nail for the radius and ulna without interlocking capability and is available in 4.0-mm and 5.0-mm diameters. Rather than interlocking, it has an interference fit design with a star-shaped cross-section to provide rotational control. Furthermore, it has a threaded cap that is designed to prevent shortening. The Stainless Steel Taper nail (Biomet, Warsaw, IN, USA) is a straight nail with interlocking screws at the insertion end of the nail and a unique interlocking device at the far end of the nail. This fixator is essentially a small internal clamp with a set screw that surrounds the nail and prevents shortening and rotation. The technique for this nail does allow for contouring of the radial nail, if necessary, to accommodate the bow.

SURGICAL TECHNIQUE

Preoperative planning is essential to determine if nail fixation is feasible. Radiography of the contralateral forearm can help with determining length, canal diameter, and the contour of the nail (if this option is available or required with the implant used). The procedure is performed under tourniquet control. Multiple positioning options are available. Supine positioning either with a radiolucent table or with an inverted image intensifier are both good options. Lateral positioning can also be used, particularly with ulna fracture reduction and nailing. Closed nailing methods are preferable to open reduction. However, open reduction is occasionally necessary in certain cases and is an acceptable method.

A preoperative radiograph of this particular case is shown in **Fig. 5**A. Operative management was chosen to facilitate early use of the upper extremity. The instruments involved for intramedullary nailing with this particular system (Acumed) are shown in **Fig. 5**B.

The ulna entry portal is proximal at the tip of the olecranon process. A 2-cm longitudinal incision is made over the olecranon (see **Fig. 5**C). A small vertical split in the triceps insertion is than made to allow placement of the opening awl. The radius entry portal is more variable depending on the manufacturer's implant design considerations. Almost all techniques, however, use a distal insertion site approximately 5 mm proximal to the joint line. Lister's tubercle serves as the primary landmark for the radius entry point. The conventional entry point for straight implants is just ulna to Lister's tubercle; however, portals just radial to Lister's tubercle are also used.[1]

An awl or hand held reamer is used to create the entry hole, which must be beveled to facilitate a more parallel entry less likely to breach the medullary cortex (see **Fig. 5**D). Closed or open reduction of the fracture is performed using the hand reamer if possible as shown in **Fig. 5**E and 5F. Hand-held reamers are then introduced into the entire length of the canal in preparation of the final implant (see **Fig. 5**G, H). Nail length is then determined with 1 of multiple acceptable methods, most commonly done as a direct-depth measurement on a calibrated reamer when fully inserted. The nail with accessory items (insertion handle with targeting device, drill sleeve, depth gauge, and locking bolt wrench) is shown in **Fig. 5**I.

With the small diameter size of the nail, forearm nails are not cannulated. Therefore, after reaming is performed, the reduction of the fracture often has to be repeated with passage of the actual nail. The nail is then carefully passed across the fracture site and inserted just short of the subchondral bone (**Fig. 5**J, K). Fluoroscopic confirmation of length and alignment is performed before the placement of interlocking screws.

Interlocking screws (typically fully threaded self-tapping screws) are then placed freehand or with the use of an aiming guide if available (**Fig. 5**L, M, N, O). Straight nails must be bent to match anatomic curves before insertion, so a sound understanding of the particular implant being used is essential during preoperative planning.

PITFALLS

As with any intramedullary nailing procedure, a narrow canal diameter can prevent insertion of intramedullary implants. Therefore, preoperative planning is essential to prevent this potential problem. Proximal interlocking screws can place the posterior interosseous nerve in danger if inserted too anteriorly. Ensuring that a parallel entry point is obtained in the radius is crucial to prevent protruding through the cortex or splitting the distal fragment.[1]

RESULTS AND COMPLICATIONS USING INTERLOCKING NAILS

Interlocking nails have been developed specifically for the forearm to avoid problems with poor control of rotation and axial length seen with unlocked

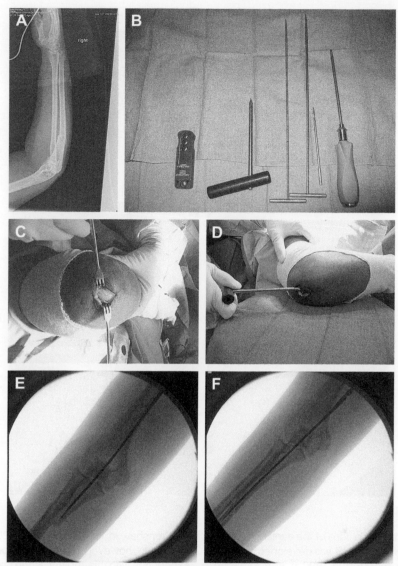

Fig. 5. Intramedullary nailing of the ulna for a minimally displaced, segmental ulna fracture in a polytraumatized patient. (*A*) A pre-operative radiograph in a polytraumatized patient demonstrates a minimally displaced segmental ulnar diaphyseal fracture. (*B*) Basic instruments required for forearm intramedullary nailing using the acumed system. From *left* to *right*: Targeting device for locking screws, opening awl, 3.0 and 3.7 mm hand reamers, drill bit for screws, screwdriver. (*C*) A 2 cm longitudinal incision is made over the olecranon process. The triceps insertion is split in line with the tendinous fibers. In this photo, the patient's head is to the left and feet are to the right. The elbow is flexed and shoulder is abducted 90 degrees. (*D*) The insertion awl is placed centrally on the olecranon and directed in line with the proximal ulna. In this case, the elbow rests and is on the inverted c-arm fluoroscope. (*E*) An AP intraoperative fluoroscopic image demonstrates insertion of the hand reamer before reduction of the fracture. (*F*) Hand reamerpassed across the fracture site after fracture reduction. (*G*) Initial hand reamer in place. (*H*) Lateral fluoroscopic image demonstrating hand reamer in place with proper portal placement proximally. (*I*) Intramedullary nail with insertion handle and targeting device for screws. Trochar and drill sleeve is seen in the bottom right corner of the photo. This insertion bolt wrench and depth gauge are seen in the top right of the photo. (*J*) Insertion of intramedullary nail. (*K*) Insertion of intramedullary nail on lateral fluoroscopic imaging. (*L*) Targeting device for proximal interlocking screw placement. (*M*), (*N*), (*O*) Intraoperative fluoroscopic images showing final position of implant and fracture alignment.

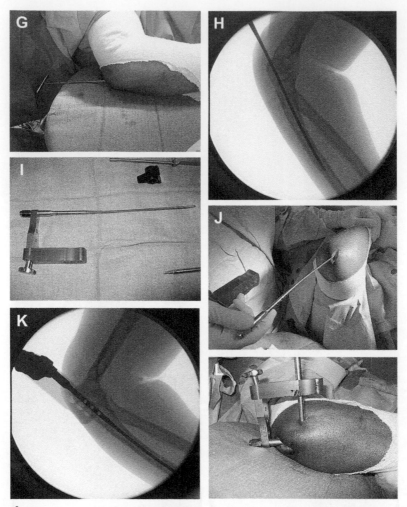

Fig. 5. (*continued*)

intramedullary methods. One of the earlier developments of an interlocking nail was developed by Lefevre and initially reported in 1990.[27] In a separate series, 20 subjects who underwent interlocked ulnar nailing using the Lefevre nail was reported in 1992.[28] Fractures included completely displaced ulnar fractures and fractures of the radius and ulna. The Lefevre nail was a 6-mm nail designed for fixation in the ulna with proximal and distal locking. In this series, closed reduction was performed with reamed intramedullary nailing up to 6.5 mm. Radius fractures were fixed with either Kirschner wires or a plate in 1 case. All fractures healed with functional results rated as 20% excellent, 70% good, and 10% fair. Nine subjects were treated with either supplemental brace or plaster cast external support. It was noted that most of the cases in this series were performed by residents and fellows, a suggestion of the simplicity of this method.

Interlocked nailing using the Foresight forearm nailing system was initially developed and reported by Crenshaw in 1999 and again in 2002.[29,30] Other surgeons, however, have also reported on their experience with this implant. Hong and colleagues[31] treated 18 subjects with 32 displaced forearm fractures from industrial accidents, motor vehicle crashes, and falls with the Foresight implants. Eight subjects also had open fractures that were treated with standard debridement procedures. The Foresight nail is available in 4.0-mm and 5.0-mm diameters and is contoured by the surgeon to match patients' anatomy. Closed nailing was done when possible with open reduction done in certain cases when necessary. Bone grafting using medullary reamings was performed in cases in which open reduction was performed. Postoperative splinting was performed in cases with secure rigid fixation and long arm casting with neutral forearm rotation was performed if fracture fixation was not secure. All fractures healed without additional procedures at an average time of 10 weeks for cases in which closed reduction was performed and 15 weeks in

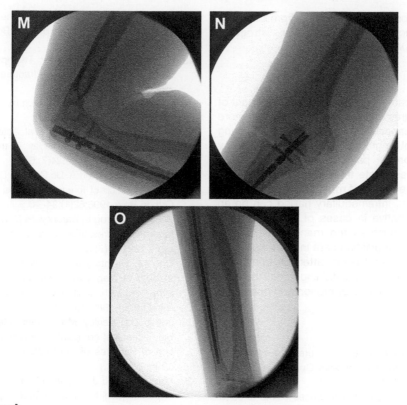

Fig. 5. (*continued*)

cases involving open reduction. Functional outcome measurements yielded a mean DASH score of 19 (range 4–72) indicating a mild to moderate impairment. Using the rating system of Grace and Eversmann, there were 13 excellent, 3 acceptable, and 2 unacceptable results. However, the incidence of complications was 22%. One synostosis occurred in a subject with closed head injury and high-energy trauma. Two distal locking screws in the ulnar nails backed out causing wrist pain and requiring removal. There was a 12.5% infection rate that was essentially caused by superficial infections in patients requiring open reductions.

Fixation of forearm fractures using the Foresight system was also reported by Weckbach in 32 subjects with forearm fractures.[32] Single bone and bone fractures were included in this study with a total of 23 ulnar nails and 17 radius nails. Union was 82% with 1 case of nonunion, 2 delayed unions, 2 cases of synostosis, and no infections. Average time to healing was 4.4 months. Full range of motion was seen in 86% of subjects and the mean DASH score was 13.7. There were no instances of implant failure or loosening except for 1 case of a broken screw. Mention was made of the technical difficulties with freehand distal interlocking and the available instrumentation for distal interlocking.

Alternative interlocking systems, such as the Acumed radius and ulna nails, have interlocking screws only at the insertion end (ie, proximal for ulna nails and distal for radius nails). This nail is available in prebent left-side and right-side specific shapes in 3.0-mm and 3.6-mm diameters and is also inserted after hand reaming to the appropriate size. Lee and colleagues[33] reported on 38 forearm fractures (18 radius, 20 ulna) that were treated with the Acumed interlocking nail system. Closed nailing was performed under fluoroscopic guidance and long arm cast immobilization was performed and bivalved postoperatively. This cast was changed to a hinged elbow brace with the forearm in neutral at the first postoperative visit. Elbow motion in the brace was performed for 6 weeks, after which the brace was removed. Average time to union was 14 weeks with only 1 case of nonunion in a subject with an open comminuted ulna fracture. There were no cases of deep infection or radioulnar synostosis. Functional results using the rating system of Grace and Eversmann yielded 81% excellent, 11% good, and 7% acceptable with mean DASH scores of 15 points.

Complications cited in the literature include radio-ulnar synostosis (especially in fractures of the radius and ulna at the same level), transient posterior interosseous nerve palsy (from interlocking screw placement), nail migration, iatrogenic fractures, malunion, and nonunion.

SUMMARY

The use of intramedullary nails in the treatment of forearm fractures has proven successful in more recent years, especially with the use of interlocking nails to control length and rotation. As with many procedures, proper patient selection cannot be overemphasized. Plate fixation remains the gold standard for treatment of most adult forearm fractures. However, intramedullary nailing can be an excellent alternative in cases of extensive soft-tissue injuries, such as the mangled or burned extremity. Other indications are in pathologic and segmental fractures. Special attention to surgical techniques, such as maintaining radial bow, is essential to prevent loss of motion and nonunion.

REFERENCES

1. Crenshaw AH, Perez EA. Fractures of the shoulder, arm, and forearm. Campbell's Operative Orthopaedics 3:3371–460.
2. Bagley C. Fracture of both bones of the forearm. Study of two hundred cases. Surg Gynecol Obstet 1928;42:95–102.
3. Bolton H, Quinlan AG. The conservative treatment of fractures of the shaft of the radius and ulna in adults. Lancet 1952;2(6737):700–5.
4. Hughston JC. Fracture of the distal radial shaft: mistakes in management. J Bone Joint Surg 1957; 39(2):249.
5. Evans EM. Rotational deformity in the treatment of fractures of both bones of the forearm. J Bone Joint Surg 1945;27(3):373.
6. Smith H, Sage FP. Medullary fixation of forearm fractures. J Bone Joint Surg 1957;39(1):91.
7. Anderson L, Sisk D, Tooms R, et al. Compression-plate fixation in acute diaphyseal fractures of the radius and ulna. J Bone Joint Surg 1975;57(3):287.
8. Chapman M, Gordon J, Zissimos A. Compression-plate fixation of acute fractures of the diaphyses of the radius and ulna. J Bone Joint Surg 1989;71(2):159.
9. Schöne G. Zur behandlung von vorderarmfrakturen mit bolzung. Münch Med Wochenschr 1913;60: 2327 [in German].
10. Rush L, Rush H. A reconstruction operation for comminuted fracture of the upper third of the ulna. Am J Surg 1937;38:332.
11. Hall R, Bugg E, Vitolo R. Intramedullary fixation of fractures of the forearm. South Med J 1952; 45(9):814.
12. Sage FP. Medullary fixation of fractures of the forearm: a study of the medullary canal of the radius

13. Ritchey SJ, Richardson JP, Thompson MS. Rigid medullary fixation of forearm fractures. South Med J 1958;51(7):852.
14. Street DM. Intramedullary forearm nailing. Clin Orthop 1986;212:219.
15. Aho A, Nieminen S, Salo U, et al. Antebrachium fractures: rush pin fixation today in the light of late results. J Trauma 1984;24(7):604.
16. Moerman J, Lenaert A, De Coninck D, et al. Intramedullary fixation of forearm fractures in adults. Acta Orthop Belg 1996;62(1):34–40.
17. Winckler S, Brug E, Baranowski D. Bundle nailing of forearm fractures. Indications and results. Unfallchirurgie 1991;94(7):335–41.
18. Ono M, Bechtold J, Merkow R, et al. Rotational stability of diaphyseal fractures of the radius and ulna fixed with Rush pins and/or fracture bracing. Clin Orthop 1989;240:236.
19. Jones DJ, Henley MB, Schemitsch EH, et al. A biomechanical comparison of two methods of fixation of fractures of the forearm. J Orthop Trauma 1995;9(3):198.
20. Martin W, Field J, Kulkarni M. Intramedullary nailing of pathological forearm fractures. Injury 2002;33(6): 530–2.
21. Hidaka S, Gustilo R. Refracture of bones of the forearm after plate removal. J Bone Joint Surg 1984; 66(8):1241.
22. Rosson J, Shearer JR. Refracture after the removal of plates from the forearm. An avoidable complication. J Bone Joint Surg 1991;73(3):415.
23. Christensen NO. Kuntscher intramedullary reaming and nail fixation for nonunion of the forearm. Clin Orthop 1976;116:215.
24. Visna P, Beitl E, Kocis J, et al. Intramedullary nail use for corrective surgery of diaphyseal forearm fractures. Scr Med 2009;(2).
25. Hong G, Cong-Feng L, Hui-Peng S, et al. Treatment of diaphyseal forearm nonunions with interlocking intramedullary nails. Clin Orthop 2006;450:186.
26. McLaren AC, Hedley A, Magee F. The effect of intramedullary rod stiffness on fracture healing. Paper presented at the 6th Annual meeting of the OTA, Toronto, October, 1990.
27. Lefevre C, Nen D, Le O, et al. L' enclouage verrouill'e de l'ulna: principles et Resultats. SICOT Meeting Abstracts. Montreal (Canada), September 9, 1990.
28. De Pedro JA, Garcia-Navarette F, De Lucas FG, et al. Internal fixation of ulnar fractures by locking nail. Clin Orthop 1992;283:81.
29. Hasty C, Crenshaw A. Intramedullary nailing of diaphyseal forearm fractures in adults. 66th Annual Meeting Proceedings [abstract]. Am Acad Orthop Surg, February 4–7, 1999;312.

30. Crenshaw AH, Zinar DM, Pickering RM. Intramedullary nailing of forearm fractures. Instr Course Lect 2002;51:279–89.

31. Hong G, Cong-Feng L, Chang-Qing Z, et al. Internal fixation of diaphyseal fractures of the forearm by interlocking intramedullary nail: short-term results in eighteen patients. J Orthop Trauma 2005;19(6):384.

32. Weckbach A, Blattert TR, Weißer C. Interlocking nailing of forearm fractures. Arch Orthop Trauma Surg 2006;126(5):309–15.

33. Lee YH, Lee SK, Chung MS, et al. Interlocking contoured intramedullary nail fixation for selected diaphyseal fractures of the forearm in adults. J Bone Joint Surg 2008;90(9):1891.

Radial Head Arthroplasty

James T. Monica, MD,
Chaitanya S. Mudgal, MD, MS (Orth), MCh (Orth)*

KEYWORDS

- Radial head • Fracture • Arthroplasty

Radial head fractures are relatively common and found in approximately 20% of all elbow trauma.[1] Radial head arthroplasty is indicated in the treatment of radial head or neck fractures when comminution precludes stable internal fixation of an unstable forearm or elbow. Radial head resection is another treatment option for comminuted radial head fractures; however, it may be associated with delayed complications, including pain, instability, proximal radial translation, ulnohumeral osteoarthrosis, decreased strength, and cubitus valgus.[1–3] In comminuted fractures, radial head resection should be avoided in the presence of lateral ulnar collateral complex injury and possible interosseous membrane injury. In such situations, radial head arthroplasty is a reliable alternative to restore radiocapitellar contact, which functions as an important stabilizer of the elbow and forearm articulations.[4] Several different arthroplasty options exist, including metal unipolar and bipolar radial head implants. This article reviews the literature related to the indications, advantages, disadvantages, techniques, and outcomes of various arthroplasty options.

ANATOMY

The articular surfaces of the radiocapitellar joint are congruent and contribute osseous stability to the elbow. The radial head is an important primary stabilizer to longitudinal stress and a secondary stabilizer against valgus stress to the elbow. The concave surface of the radial head articulates with the hemispheric-shaped capitellum and the radial head rim articulates with the lesser sigmoid notch. Articular cartilage covers the concave surface as well as an arc of approximately 280° of the rim.[5] The radial head is not perfectly circular and is variably offset from the axis of the neck, which has important implications in radial head reconstruction. The primary stabilizer to varus stress consists of the lateral collateral ligament complex (LCL). The LCL complex consists of four components: radial collateral ligament, the lateral ulnar collateral ligament, the annular ligament, and the accessory collateral ligament. The lateral ulnar collateral ligament is one of the primary elbow constraints because it provides varus and posterolateral stability by its insertion distal to the posterior attachment of the annular ligament on the crista supinatoris.[6]

INDICATIONS

The indications for use of a metallic radial head prosthesis include an acute comminuted fracture in which satisfactory reduction and stable fixation cannot be obtained. Radial head replacement may also be considered in patients with complex elbow injuries that involve greater than 30% of the articular rim of the radial head, which cannot be reconstructed.[7] Data by Ring and colleagues[4] suggest that open reduction and internal fixation are best reserved for minimally comminuted fractures with 3 or fewer articular fragments. Patients who present in a delayed manner with persistent pain and instability from radial head primary resections, malunions, or posttraumatic arthritis or after complex elbow fracture-dislocations involving the radial head are also candidates for radial head arthroplasty.

Hand and Upper Extremity Surgery Service, Department of Orthopaedic Surgery, Massachusetts General Hospital, Harvard Medical School, 55 Fruit Street, Yawkey Center, Suite 2100, Boston, MA 02114, USA
* Corresponding author.
E-mail address: cmudgal@partners.org

Hand Clin 26 (2010) 403–410
doi:10.1016/j.hcl.2010.04.008
0749-0712/10/$ – see front matter. Published by Elsevier Inc.

Active infection is a contraindication to radial head arthroplasty.[7] Radial head arthroplasty may also be contraindicated in patients with advanced radiocapitellar arthrosis where the capitellum is destroyed or devoid of any articular cartilage.

AVAILABLE IMPLANTS

Several current implant options are available. Major differences between current implants include unipolar versus bipolar heads, cemented versus cementless stems, and monoblock versus modular designs (**Table 1**).

The Ascension Modular Radial Head (Ascension Orthopedics, Austin, TX, USA) is a unipolar head (**Fig. 1**). The radial head resection guide has two different levels depending on the amount of radial neck involved in the fracture. The implant can be assembled in situ by placing the head on the morse taper of the stem and using an offset head impactor. Multiple head/stem sizes and configurations accommodate a broad range of patient anatomy. These include 3 diameters of long and standard length heads combined with 3 different stem diameters and a long stem that mimics the proximal radial bow (**Fig. 2**). Ascension is also developing a pyrolytic carbon implant (**Fig. 3**).

The CRF II by Tornier (Saint-Ismier Cedex, France) developed by Judet and colleagues,[8] was the first radial head bipolar prosthesis. It is available in 2 head and 3 stem diameters (**Fig. 4**). The cemented stem has a 15° proximal angle and the bipolar articulation of polyethylene on cobalt chrome allows for a range of motion of 35° between the head and stem. This motion is thought to provide full radial head articulation on the capitellum throughout elbow range of motion. The set also includes a radial resection template for a precise cut.

The Evolve Modular Radial Head (Wright Medical Technology, Arlington, TN, USA) is another modular implant that allows for in situ assembly (**Fig. 5**). The system has a radial neck planer that slips over the trial stem to create a smooth contact surface on the radial neck, perpendicular to the longitudinal axis of the radial neck. An in situ assembly tool with a long lever arm is used to ensure a 2000-N assembly load is applied to secure the head on the morse tapered neck.[9]

The Katalyst by KMI (Carlsbad, CA, USA) is also a bipolar radial head system. Three radial head diameters are available and the radial head height is adjustable through a telescoping neck by increments of 2 mm to 10 mm (**Figs. 6** and **7**). The neck length is secured with screws. Two options are available for stem diameter. The bipolar articulation consists of a cobalt chrome ball and an ultra–high molecular weight polyethylene socket. The articulation allows for 15° of motion between the neck and head. The modular design is suggested to allow implant insertion without disruption of the lateral ligament complex.

The Solar Radial Head Implant System (Stryker, Mahwah, NJ, USA) (**Fig. 8**) is a monoblock cobalt chrome implant that is available in 5 sizes with heads available in 2 diameters. This implant is available only for cement fixation.

The Swanson Titanium Radial Head implant (Wright Medical, Arlington, TX, USA) (**Fig. 9**) features a titanium implant with nitrogen ion implantation for increased surface hardness. It has a short, wider stem to allow easier placement. Permanent fixation in the intramedullary canal is not required. The implant is available in 5 different sizes.

The ExploR® Modular Radial Head by Biomet (Warsaw, IN, USA) (**Fig. 10**) is a modular head and stem that does not require assembly before implantation, allowing for in situ replacement. Three head diameters, each with 5 different lengths (15 head options), and 5 different stem options provide for optimal patient sizing with more than 75 different combinations. There is a bond-coated stem that theoretically allows for enhanced fixation.

The rHead radial implant system by Small Bone Innovations (SBI, Morrisville, PA, USA) (**Fig. 11**) offers a modular unipolar implant with 3 different heights and diameters. There is also an extended collar to be used with distally migrated fractures of the proximal radius. The system includes a radial head resection guide that is used to cut the proximal radius at 3 different heights corresponding to the 3 different thicknesses of radial head implant available. After broaching, the stem is inserted in an arc-like fashion, facilitated by the curve of the stem that corresponds to the 15° lateral angle created by the native radial head and shaft. The head is then inserted onto the neck taper.

TECHNIQUE

The radial head may be approached through a lateral or posterior approach. Often when concomitant fractures about the elbow are present and require fixation, an extensile posterior approach is preferred. A curvilinear incision is made between the lateral condylar ridge and the midaxial line of the radial neck. Dissection through the Kocher interval between the anconeus and extensor carpi ulnaris or the Kaplan interval between the extensor carpi radialis longus and extensor digitorum communis or splitting the extensor digitorum communis, as described by

Table 1
Radial head implants

rHead (Small Bone Innovations)	Liverpool Radial Head Replacement (Biomet Merck)	Ascension (Ascension Orthopedics)	CRF II (Tornier)	Katalyst (KMI, Carlsbad, CA, USA)	Swanson Titanium Radial Head (Wright Medical Technology)	Evolve (Wright Medical Technology)
• Unipolar/ bipolar option 20° arc • Modular • 3 Head heights • 3 Head diameters • 8 Stem sizes • Porous coated stem • In situ assembly	• Unipolar • Monoblock • 15 Implant sizes • Porous coated stem	• Unipolar • Modular • 2 Head heights • 3 Head diameters • 4 Stem sizes • In situ assembly	• Bipolar—arc 35° • Modular • 4 Head diameters • 5 Stem diameters • 2 Stem lengths	• Bipolar—arc 15° • Modular • 2-mm Spacers to adjust head height up to 10 mm in situ • 3 Diameters • 2 Stem sizes	• Unipolar • Monoblock • 5 Implant sizes	• Unipolar • Modular • 15 Head sizes • 10 Stem sizes • In situ assembly

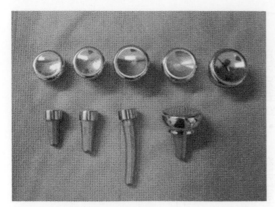

Fig. 1. The Ascension Modular Radial Head (Ascension Orthopedics, Austin, TX, USA).

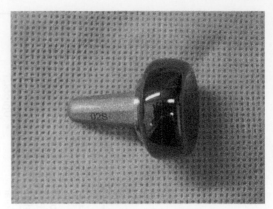

Fig. 3. The Ascension Modular Radial Head, pyrolytic carbon (Ascension Orthopedics, Austin, TX, USA).

Hotchkiss, may be performed.[10] Care should be taken to protect the LCL complex posteriorly when using the Kocher approach as well as protecting the posterior interosseous nerve when using the Kaplan approach.[11] All the ligamentous origin may be taken down anterior to a line bisecting the articular surface of the capitellum from a lateral vantage point.[10] A cadaver study of radial head plating by Tornetta and colleagues[12] reported that in only 1 (2%) of 50 arms did the posterior interosseous nerve lie directly on the radius. The average distance from the radial head to the origin of the posterior interosseous nerve was 1.2 ± 1.9 mm, with the takeoff being proximal to the radial head in 31 cases. The muscular branch to the extensor carpi radialis longus was located 7.1 ± 1.8 mm from the radial head.[12] Inspection of the LCL complex should be performed. The elbow capsule and annular ligament should be incised in line with the posterior margin of the extensor carpi ulanris. The capsule can also be incised in a ligamentous-sparing Z capsulotomy, as described by Bain.[7] The capsule

is elevated off the anterior distal humerus and more of the radiocapitellar joint may be exposed by elevating the origin of the brachioradialis. At all times, every effort is made to keep the forearm pronated and vigorous traction on the anterior soft tissues is avoided so as to reduce the possibility of any iatrogenic injury to the posterior interosseous nerve. Retraction is best done with sutures placed in the anterior capsule. Exposure provided by retractors, such as the Hohmann retractor placed anteriorly around the radial head or neck, is excellent; however, the authors recommend against their use to prevent any form of traction on the posterior interosseous nerve. Should the radial head need to be delivered into the wound for enhanced exposure, placing a small Hohmann

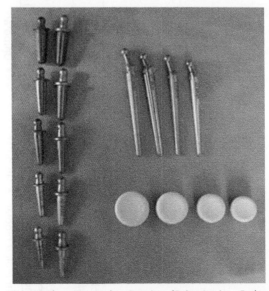

Fig. 4. The CRF II by Tornier (Saint-Ismier Cedex, France).

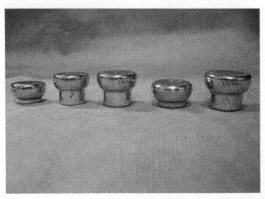

Fig. 2. The Ascension Modular Radial Head (Ascension Orthopedics, Austin, TX, USA).

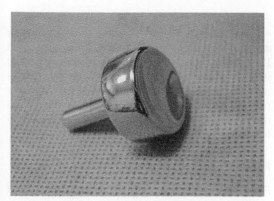

Fig. 5. The Evolve Modular Radial Head (Wright Medical Technology, Arlington, TN, USA).

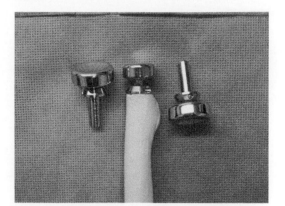

Fig. 7. The Katalyst by KMI (Carlsbad, CA, USA).

retractor gently on the dorsal surface of the head is helpful in elevating the radial head into the wound.[10]

Once the radial head is exposed, the degree of comminution is assessed and a decision made whether or not to attempt fixation or replacement. Although current implants and techniques for internal fixation of small articular fractures have made it possible to repair most fractures of the radial head, data by Ring and colleagues[4] suggest that open reduction and internal fixation are best reserved for minimally comminuted fractures with 3 or fewer articular fragments. Goals of implant placement are to replicate the native radial head anatomy as closely as possible with special attention paid to radial head size and height.[13] Multiple biomechanical studies have demonstrated the importance of accurate radial head sizing.[14–16] The fractured head should be reassembled as close to anatomically as possible, and an appropriate head size is selected. Care should be taken to avoid overstuffing the radiocapitellar joint because it has been associated with radiocapitellar wear and erosion.[16] The longitudinal height of the prosthetic head is selected based on the

height of the radial head fragments with use of a trial prosthesis for comparison. If comminution of the radial head prohibits accurate measurement of length, the lateral edge of the coronoid process at the proximal portion of the lesser sigmoid notch may be used as a landmark. Doornberg and colleagues[17] demonstrated in CT scans of 17 elbows that the native radial head lies an average of 0.9 mm distal to the proximal margin of the sigmoid notch. In general, it is preferable for the diameter and the thickness of the prosthesis to be slightly undersized.[18] A prosthesis with a diameter that is too large points load on the margins of the sigmoid notch, whereas a prosthesis that is too small points load on the sigmoid notch.[19] A radial head with an incorrect diameter also has a cam effect, which produces abnormal loading on the capitellum. Insertion of a radial head that is too short contributes to radiocapitellar instability.[19]

A neck planer may be used to create a smooth contact with the radial head implant. The radial neck is then reamed to remove cancellous bone and reaming is complete when cortical bone is reached. In most contemporary radial head replacement systems, a stem size that is one

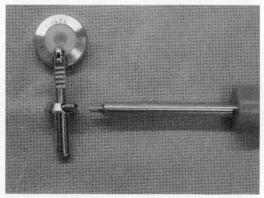

Fig. 6. The Katalyst by KMI (Carlsbad, CA, USA).

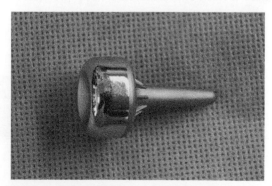

Fig. 8. The Solar Radial Head Implant System (Stryker, Mahwah, NJ, USA).

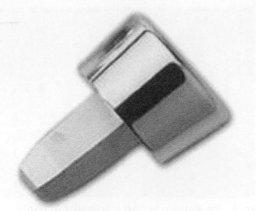

Fig. 9. The Swanson Titanium Radial Head implant. (*Courtesy of* Wright Medical Technology, Arlington, Texas; with permission.)

size smaller than the final reamer is selected. The fit between the stem and radial neck is loose in most implants to allow the annular ligament to guide radiocapitellar articular contact rather than the fixed stem. A loose fitting stem compensates for the shortcomings of a well-fixed stem attempting to restore the variable radial head anatomy with an elliptical head and an offset neck. Inserting the stem may be difficult if the LCL is intact. An effective way to facilitate prosthesis insertion is to place a retractor under the radial neck and lever the proximal part of the radius anteriorly and laterally away from the capitellum.[18]

Once the radial head implant is placed, elbow range of motion and stability are tested. Formal assessment of elbow stability as described by Bain includes stress testing with the elbow in 30° flexion and the forearm pronated.[7] In this position, narrowing of the radiocapitellar joint by 2 mm with valgus stress testing is indicative of loss of integrity of the anterior band of the ulnar collateral ligament. Transosseus sutures should be used for stabilization of the LCL with the elbow in 30° flexion and the forearm in full pronation.[19]

Beingessner and colleagues[20] reported in a biomechanical study that varus-valgus laxity was corrected after radial head arthroplasty and LUCL repair but not after radial head arthroplasty without ligament repair. They noted only a small amount of instability in elbows with disrupted medial collateral ligaments after radial head replacement, which they attributed to compensatory stabilization from the biceps and brachialis.

POSTOPERATIVE REHABILITATION

Postoperatively, early range of motion is important to ensure a successful outcome. Patients begin formal rehabilitative therapy for active and active assisted range of motion within the first week after surgery. Stability of the surgical wound must be confirmed before instituting rehabilitation. Splinting between rehabilitation exercises is based on the particular elbow injury encountered and, in most circumstances, is discontinued within the first 2 to 3 weeks after surgery. Strengthening is initiated 6 weeks after surgery.

OUTCOMES
Unipolar Implants

Most contemporary radial head implants are made of cobalt-chromium or titanium. Silicone implants used in the past have been found to provide inadequate stability and in most circumstances tend to break down over time causing synovitis and its sequelae.[21,22] Metallic implants have been shown to reproduce the loads across the elbow more closely than silicone implants.[19] Pyrolytic carbon is now being considered as an implant material in radial head implants. Theoretic advantages include an elastic modulus close to cortical bone, favorable wear characteristics,[23] and less wear damage to cartilage in canines.[24]

The stems of unipolar implants are loose fitting or fixed stems. Fixed stems require a close approximation to native anatomy to achieve joint

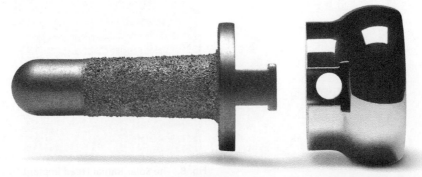

Fig. 10. The ExploR® Modular Radial Head by Biomet. (*Courtesy of* Biomet Orthopedics, Warsaw, IN; with permission.)

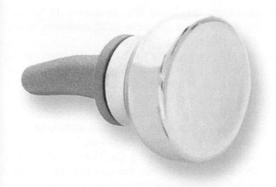

Fig. 11. The rHead by Small Bone Innovations. (*Courtesy of* SBI, Morrisville, Pennsylvania; with permission.)

congruity. It is believed that smooth stems allow the radial head implant to settle in an anatomic position during range of motion and act as a spacer arthroplasty.

Grewal and colleagues[25] reported 12 excellent, 4 good, 6 fair, and 2 poor results in 26 patients with Mason type III fractures at an average of 25 months after fracture. Harrington and colleagues[26] reported 12 excellent, 4 good, 2 fair, and 2 poor results an average of 12 years after surgery in 14 Mason type IV (comminuted fracture dislocations), 3 Monteggia fracture dislocations, 2 medial ligament tears associated with radial head fractures, and 1 Mason type II radial neck and coronoid fracture. Eighty percent of the patients had good to excellent overall modified Mayo Clinic functional rating index system scores.[27] All had radiologic lucency around the stem. Eleven patients showed no evidence of degenerative joint disease. After an average of 58 months, mild changes were observed in 6 patients, moderate changes in 2, and severe changes in only 1 patient with a combined radial head fracture and medial ligament tear.[26]

The majority of patients with loose fitting stems have radiographic lucency around the stem at follow-up as reported by Doornberg and colleagues.[28] They followed 27 patients, 11 with Mason type II and 16 with Mason type III fractures, for an average of 40 months and reported average range of motion of −20° extension, 131° flexion, 73° pronation, and 57° supination. Ten radial head fractures were associated with a posterior fracture-dislocation of the olecranon and a coronoid fracture; 16 were associated with a complete posterior dislocation of the elbow, and 1 was associated with an MCL rupture and subluxation. Twenty of 27 patients had excellent results on Mayo Elbow Performance Index.[27] Seven patients had subsequent operations to treat residual instability, heterotopic ossification, elbow contracture, ulnar neuropathy, or a misplaced screw. The

implants were intentionally inserted loosely to accommodate for the inevitable differences between the implant and native radial head.[28] In a study of 25 patients, 10 with Mason type III and 15 with Mason type IV injuries, with an average of 39 months' follow-up, Moro and colleagues[29] reported lucency around the stem without subsidence as being the norm.

Knight and colleagues[30] reported a reliable restoration of stability and prevention of proximal radial head migration after unipolar metal prosthesis in 31 patients at an average of 4.5 years' follow-up; 68% of the radial head fractures were associated with elbow dislocations. They noted a low complication rate and only 2 implants were removed for aseptic loosening.

Bipolar Implants

Judet and colleagues[8] reported results of a floating prosthesis in 12 patients at an average of 2 years' follow-up. Of 5 patients treated acutely, 3 had excellent results and 2 were classified as having a good result. Seven patients were treated with radial head arthroplasty after failed open reduction internal fixation. There were 1 excellent, 4 good, and 3 fair results. Holmenschlager and colleagues[27,31] reported on 16 bipolar prostheses with a 19-month follow-up. There were 2 excellent, 12 good, 1 fair, and 1 poor result using the evaluation system of Morrey.[27] Complications included 1 transient radial nerve palsy, 1 reflex sympathetic dystrophy, and 1 asymptomatic loosening.[31] Pomianowski and colleagues[14] performed a cadaver study that showed that a bipolar radial head prosthesis can be as effective as a solid monoblock prosthesis in restoring valgus stability in a medial collateral ligament–deficient elbow.

SUMMARY

Reported clinical outcomes of metallic radial head arthroplasty indicate that radial head arthroplasty is a reasonable treatment option to offer patients with comminuted radial head fractures in which stable internal fixation is not possible in an unstable forearm or elbow. Careful attention to surgical anatomy and technique is crucial to ensuring a good outcome. Several implant options and techniques of implantation are available to orthopedic surgeons to help optimize patient outcome.

REFERENCES

1. Herbertsson P, Josefsson PO, Hasserius R, et al. Fractures of the radial head and neck treated with radial head excision. J Bone Joint Surg Am 2004; 86:1925–30.

2. Morrey BF, Tanaka S, An KN. Valgus stability of the elbow: a definition of primary and secondary constraints. Clin Orthop Relat Res 1991;265:187–95.

3. Ikeda M, Oka Y. Function after early radial head resection for fracture: a retrospective evaluation of 15 patients followed for 3–18 years. Acta Orthop Scand 2000;71:191–4.

4. Ring D, Quintero J, Jupiter JB. Open reduction and internal fixation of fractures of the radial head. J Bone Joint Surg Am 2002;84:1811–5.

5. Bryce CD, Armstrong AD. Anatomy and biomechanics of the elbow. Orthop Clin North Am 2008; 39:141–54.

6. Johnson JA, King GJ. Anatomy and biomechanics of the elbow. In: Williams GR, Yamaguchi K, Ramsey ML, et al, editors. Shoulder and elbow arthroplasty. Philadelphia: Lippincott Williams and Wilkins; 2005. p. 279–96.

7. Bain GI, Ashwood N, Baird R, et al. Management of mason type-III radial head fractures with a titanium prosthesis, ligament repair, and early mobilization. J Bone Joint Surg Am 2005;87:136–47.

8. Judet T, Garreau de Loubresse C, Piriou P, et al. A floating prosthesis for radial-head fractures. J Bone Joint Surg Br 1996;78:244–9.

9. Technique guide from Wright Medical Technology, Inc. Evolve modular radial head: surgical technique guide. November 2002.

10. Hotchkiss RN. Displaced fractures of the radial head: internal fixation or excision. J Am Acad Orthop Surg 1997;5:1–10.

11. Morrey BF. Surgical exposures of the elbow. In: Morrey BF, editor. The elbow and its disorders. 2nd edition. Philadephia: W.B. Sanders; 1993. p. 139–66.

12. Tornetta P, Hochwald N, Bono C, et al. Anatomy of the posterior interosseous nerve in relation to fixation of the radial head. Clin Orthop Relat Res 1997;345: 215–8.

13. King GJW. Management of comminuted radial head fractures with replacement arthroplasty. Hand Clin 2004;20:429–41.

14. Pomianowski S, Morrey BF, Neale PG, et al. Contribution of monoblock and bipolar radial head prostheses to valgus stability of the elbow. J Bone Joint Surg Am 2001;83:1829–34.

15. Smith GR, Hotchkiss RN. Radial head and neck fractures: anatomic guidelines for proper placement of internal fixation. J Shoulder Elbow Surg 1996; 5(2 Pt 1):113–7.

16. Van Glabbeek F, Van Riet RP, Baumfeld JA, et al. Detrimental effects of overstuffing or understuffing with a radial head replacement in the medial collateral-ligament deficient elbow. J Bone Joint Surg Am 2004;86:2629–35.

17. Doornberg JN, Linzel DS, Zurakowski D, et al. Reference points for radial head prosthesis size. J Hand Surg Am 2006;31:53–7.

18. Ring D, King G. Radial head arthroplasty with a modular metal spacer to treat acute traumatic elbow instability: surgical technique. J Bone Joint Surg Am 2008;90:63–73.

19. King GJ, Zarzour ZD, Rath DA, et al. Metallic radial head arthroplasty improves valgus stability of the elbow. Clin Orthop 1999;368:114–25.

20. Beingessner DM, Dunning CE, Gordon KD, et al. The effect of radial head excision and arthroplasty on elbow kinematics and stability. J Bone Joint Surg Am 2004;86:1730–9.

21. Morrey BF, Askew L, Chao EY. Silastic prosthetic replacement for the radial head. J Bone Joint Surg Am 1981;63:454–8.

22. Worsing RA Jr, Engber WD, Lange TA. Reactive synovitis from particulate silastic. J Bone Joint Surg Am 1982;64:581–5.

23. Strzepa P, Klawitter J. Ascension pyrocarbon hemisphere wear testing against bone. Poster No. 0897, 51st Annual Meeting of the Orthopaedic Research Society. Washington, DC, February 2005.

24. Cook SD, Thomas KA, Kester MA. Wear characteristics of the canine acetabulum against different femoral prosthesis. J Bone Joint Surg Br 1989; 71(2):189–97.

25. Grewal R, MacDermid JC, Faber KJ, et al. Comminuted radial head fractures treated with a modular metallic radial head arthroplasty: study of outcomes. J Bone Joint Surg Am 2006;88:2192–200.

26. Harrington IJ, Sekyi-Otu A, Barrington TW, et al. The functional outcome with metallic radial head implants in the treatment of unstable elbow fractures: a long-term review. J Trauma 2001;50: 46–52.

27. Morrey BF. The elbow and its disorders. 2nd edition. Philadelphia: Saunders; 1993.

28. Doornberg JN, Parisien R, van Duijn J, et al. Radial head arthroplasty with a modular metal spacer to treat traumatic elbow instability. J Bone Joint Surg Am 2007;89:1075–80.

29. Moro JK, Werier J, MacDermid JC, et al. Arthroplasty with a metal radial head for unreconstructible fractures of the radial head. J Bone Joint Surg Am 2001;83:1202–11.

30. Knight DJ, Rymaszewski LA, Amis AA, et al. Primary replacement of the fractured radial head with a metal prosthesis. J Bone Joint Surg Br 1993;75:572–6.

31. Holmenschlager F, Halm JP, Winckler S. [Fresh fractures of the radial head: results with the Judet prosthesis]. Rev Chir Orthop Reparatrice Appar Mot 2002;88:387–97 [in French].

Use of Orthogonal or Parallel Plating Techniques to Treat Distal Humerus Fractures

Joshua M. Abzug, MD[a],*, Phani K. Dantuluri, MD[b,c,d]

KEYWORDS

- Distal humerus fractures • Parallel plating
- Orthogonal plating • Open reduction and internal fixation

Fractures of the distal humerus account for 2% to 6% of all fractures.[1] These fractures occur in a bimodal age distribution, with fractures in younger patients occurring as a result of high-energy mechanisms and fragility fractures occurring in the elderly as a result of low-energy falls.[2] The subsequent fracture pattern present may be extra-articular (AO type A), partial articular (AO type B), or complete articular (AO type C.)[3] Other classification systems used are the Jupiter and Mehne[4] system, which is based on fracture patterns observed intraoperatively, and the system proposed by Davies and Stanley, which combines the aforementioned classifications into one system.[5] Whatever system is used, it is important to pay particular attention to the mechanism of injury, the condition of the soft tissues, the bone quality, and lastly the age and physical demands of patients.

All of these fractures represent a challenge to the surgeon because of the distal location and predilection toward articular involvement. Because of these issues, multiple treatment strategies have emerged with the majority of current recommendations including open reduction and internal fixation (ORIF.) ORIF of the fracture allows the surgeon to restore anatomic alignment of the fracture fragments and permit early range-of-motion exercises that may aid in the return of a functional range of motion of the elbow postoperatively. Different methods of internal fixation of the fracture fragments have evolved over time in an attempt to best restore anatomic alignment of the distal humerus, given its complex anatomy while also providing stable fixation to permit early rehabilitation of the injured extremity.

The distal humerus is composed of a medial and lateral column with a central area of thin weaker bone. This central area, the coronoid and olecranon fossae, is present to facilitate elbow flexion and extension by allowing a space for the olecranon tip to articulate, while also providing bony stability. However, this central area has been shown to be particularly thin in patients with osteopenia, thus making it a common site of

Dr Abzug is a hand surgery fellow, Thomas Jefferson University Hospital, The Philadelphia Hand Center, Philadelphia, PA.

[a] The Philadelphia Hand Center, Department of Orthopaedic Surgery, Thomas Jefferson University Hospital, 834 Chestnut Street, Suite G114, Philadelphia, PA, USA
[b] Department of Orthopaedics, Emory University Midtown Hospital, 550 Peachtree Street Northeast, Atlanta, GA, USA
[c] Department of Orthopaedics, Atlanta Medical Center, 303 Parkway Drive Northeast, Atlanta, GA, USA
[d] Department of Orthopaedics, Resurgens Orthopaedics, 550 Peachtree Street, 19th Floor, Atlanta, GA, USA
* Corresponding author. The Philadelphia Hand Center, Department of Orthopaedic Surgery, Thomas Jefferson University Hospital, 834 Chestnut Street, Suite G114, Philadelphia, PA.
E-mail address: jabzug1@yahoo.com

Hand Clin 26 (2010) 411–421
doi:10.1016/j.hcl.2010.05.008

involvement with fractures of the distal humerus.[6] It is essential that this area be reconstructed to restore diaphyseal-metaphyseal contact to provide the most stability and allow for the best healing potential.[7] Because of this unique anatomy of the distal humerus, various plates have been developed to try and provide adequate stability to the articular, metaphyseal, and diaphyseal regions of the distal humerus. These plates include Y-shaped plates, recon plates contoured to the anatomy, and recently, precontoured plates with or without locking screw capabilities.

The anatomic location to place the plates on the distal humerus has recently been debated throughout the literature with the majority of authors currently recommending at least two plates be used to provide adequate stability and allow for adequate restoration of anatomy. Orthogonal plating, otherwise known as 90-90 plating or perpendicular plating, involves placing one plate on the medial column of the distal humerus and the other plate along the posterolateral column. The concept of parallel plating involves placing one plate along the medial column of the distal humerus and the other plate along the lateral column.

ANATOMY

The elbow joint is characterized as being a hinge joint because it only has a single axis of rotation.[8] This rotation primarily occurs between the semilunar notch at the proximal part of the ulna and the trochlea at the distal end of the humerus. The trochlea is bounded on each side by a bony column, thus forming a bony construct that is analogous to a triangle. If any of the arms of the triangle are disrupted, the entire construct is weakened more than expected.[9] Therefore, it is important to ensure each arm of this bony construct has adequate fixation when performing an ORIF of the distal humerus.

The medial and lateral bony columns surrounding the trochlea have different anatomic extensions. The medial column terminates approximately 1 cm proximal to the distal end of the trochlea, whereas the lateral column extends to the distal aspect of the trochlea.[10] The anterior surface at the distal extent of lateral column is covered with articular cartilage, thus forming the capitellum.

On the anterior aspect of the distal humerus, the coronoid fossa is present just proximal to the trochlea and the radial fossa is present just proximal to the capitellum. These fossae are separated by a longitudinal bony ridge that continues distally with the lateral lip of the trochlea.[10] The

longitudinal ridge and the lateral lip of the trochlea form the anterior anatomic division between the medial and lateral columns.

On the posterior aspect of the distal humerus, the olecranon fossa is present to accommodate the tip of the olecranon when the elbow is in full extension. The distal humerus itself is quite thin between the medial and lateral columns at this level because the intramedullary canal actually tapers to an end approximately 2 to 3 cm proximal to the olecranon fossa. In fact, 6% of the population may have an actual bony defect, a septal aperture, in this area.[10]

The medial column of the distal humerus diverges from the humeral shaft at approximately a 45° angle. The proximal two-thirds of this column is made up of cortical bone, whereas the distal third is formed by the medial epicondyle, composed of cancellous bone.[11] The lateral column of the distal humerus is subtended at approximately a 20° angle in reference to the humeral shaft. The proximal half of the lateral column is composed of cortical bone, whereas the distal half is composed of cancellous bone.[10] The proximal portion is not only composed of cortical bone but also a flat and broad surface, thus making it ideal for placement of a plate.

CLASSIFICATION SCHEMES

Fractures of the distal humerus have historically been classified based on anatomic considerations. Initially these fractures were classified based on the concept that the distal end of the humerus was made up of condyles. The terms supracondylar, condylar, transcondylar, and bicondylar fractures were used.[12]

Currently, fractures of the distal humerus are more commonly described based on the previously discussed anatomic description of the columnar structure of the distal humerus, which includes describing fractures as single columnar, bicolumnar, and transcolumnar fractures. In addition, fractures can be classified based on the specific bony fragment involved (ie, trochlear, capitellar, medial epicondylar, or lateral epicondylar fractures).

Single column fractures make up 3% to 4% of distal humerus fractures and more commonly involve the lateral column.[13] These fractures involve the medial or lateral column and extend distally through the intercolumnar portion of the distal humerus.[10]

Bicolumnar fractures are the most common type of distal humerus fracture representing 5% to 62% of distal humerus fractures.[10] These fractures involve each limb of the triangle discussed earlier, thus making them extremely difficult to treat.[10] It is this difficulty that has led to the ongoing debate over which type of fracture fixation is best to provide the most rigid fixation that will facilitate rapid healing while still allowing early range of motion.

RATIONALE
Orthogonal Plating

Orthogonal plating techniques evolved after a publication by Jupiter and colleagues[14] in 1985, reporting on patients having successful outcomes with ORIF of distal humerus fractures. This retrospective series looked at 39 subjects treated with ORIF of the distal humerus and found 27 subjects to have good or excellent results. They noted that the key to surgical success was obtaining enough bony stability to permit early range of motion. This stability usually required the use of two plates, one on the medial column and the other on the lateral column.[14]

Before this report, the literature had a wide range of treatment recommendations ranging from nonoperative treatment to ORIF with limited internal fixation. These series had few numbers and used different outcome measures, thus making comparisons among various treatment methods extremely difficult.[10] Despite this, it became accepted that Kirschner-wire fixation alone did not provide adequate stability to treat bicolumnar distal humeral fractures.[15,16] In addition, Waddell and colleagues[17] have shown that elbow immobilization of 3 to 4 weeks postoperatively leads to unacceptable stiffness. One caveat to this is that if the fracture is severely comminuted and the fixation is suboptimal, it may be better to immobilize the elbow for an extended period to allow fracture union and then deal with a stiff elbow with fracture union because that may be preferable to failure of fixation and a nonunion, which may result from an attempt at early mobilization in these patients.

Based on these observations, Jupiter and colleagues established the technique of orthogonal plating to provide adequate stability of the fracture fragments to allow bony healing and early postoperative rehabilitation.

Parallel Plating

The concept of parallel plating was conceived because some surgeons thought that the described technique of orthogonal plating was not sufficient for all cases because there were some cases where orthogonal plating provided inadequate fixation of the distal fragments and not enough stability between the intraarticular distal fragments and the humeral shaft. Several authors have documented a 20% to 25% rate of unsatisfactory results following orthogonal plating of distal humerus fractures. Henley and colleagues[18] had failure of fixation in 5 of 33 subjects, whereas Letsch and colleagues[19] had failures in 5 of 88 fractures. There were failures in 3 of 57 subjects treated by Holdsworth and Mossad,[20] whereas Wildburger's series demonstrated failure in 9 of 72 fractures.[21] Additionally, Sodergard and colleagues[22] had failures in 16 of 96 fractures. When fixation does fail, it occurs at the supracondylar level.[23] This failure occurs because of suboptimal anchorage of the articular fragments to the shaft caused by the limited number and length of screws that can be placed in the distal fragments.[23]

When early motion is permitted in fractures treated without adequate stability, motion occurring at the fracture site can lead to nonunion.[24] Korner and colleagues[25] noted that 75% of malunion or nonunion cases were caused by inadequate initial fracture fixation. Alternatively, if the elbow was immobilized for a prolonged period of time to accommodate for the tenuous fixation, resultant elbow stiffness may occur.[26] An additional rationale for use of parallel plating is that longer screws can be placed from a medial to lateral direction as opposed to a screw placed through a posterolateral plate.[6] Based on these observations, the Mayo Clinic group proposed the idea of parallel plating using the principles of enhancing fixation of the distal fragments and achieving stability at the supracondylar level.[23] There are 8 technical objectives that have been described concerning parallel plating. There are 6 objectives related to distal screw insertion and 2 related to plate fixation.

With regard to distal screw insertion, each screw should pass through a plate. Additionally, each screw should engage a fragment on the opposite side that is also fixed to a plate. There should be an adequate number of screws placed in the distal fragments and each screw should be as long as possible engaging as many articular fragments as possible. Lastly, the screws should lock together by interdigitation, creating a fixed-angle structure and linking the columns together.[27] With regard to fixation of the plates, the plates should be applied allowing for compression of both columns at the supracondylar level. Lastly, the plates chosen must have enough strength and stiffness to resist breaking or bending before union occurs at the supracondylar level.[27] It was the Mayo Clinic group's belief that following these technical objectives would allow the parallel plating technique to link both columns of the distal humerus, thus providing the structural stability necessary for fracture healing. The interdigitation of the distal screws is likened to a keystone of an arch, being the structural link necessary for adequate fixation.[27] Thus, fixation of the bone fragments relies on the stability of the hardware construct rather than on screw purchase in the bone.[23]

BIOMECHANICAL ANALYSIS

The literature has had contradictory results with regard to biomechanical testing of these two techniques. Self and colleagues[28] assessed the biomechanical aspects of the two techniques using reconstruction plates and found the parallel system to be stronger and stiffer. Jacobson and colleagues[29] also assessed the biomechanical aspects of the techniques with reconstruction plates yet found the perpendicular system to be stronger. Both of these studies were performed on cadaveric bone.

Schwartz and colleagues[30] assessed nonlocking periarticular plates on composite bone and found similar biomechanical properties in both techniques. More recently, Stoffel and colleagues assessed the biomechanical principles of the techniques using locking plates. The authors used 24 humeri from fresh-frozen female cadavers and found stability was most dependent on bone quality. However, within their analysis the parallel plating system was found to have significantly higher stability in compression and external rotation and a greater ability to resist axial plastic deformation.[31]

Schuster and colleagues also used cadaveric bones to assess the biomechanical properties of various plates using the orthogonal plating technique for simulated type C2 distal humerus fractures. Their assessment included a comparison of fractures treated with conventional reconstruction plates, locking compression plates, and locking distal humerus plates. Similar to the aforementioned study by Stoffel and colleagues, this study determined that stability was dependent on bone-mineral density. When good bone quality was present, the choice of implant did not matter. However, when bone-mineral density was low ($< 420 \, \text{mg/cm}^3$) both locking plates provided superior resistance against screw loosening compared with the nonlocking conventional reconstruction plate.[32] Based on this biomechanical data the authors recommend use of locking plates for comminuted or osteopenic fractures.

SURGICAL TECHNIQUES

ORIF should be performed in fractures with any amount of significant displacement involving the articular surface because outcomes are superior to nonsurgical treatment of these fractures. The goals of ORIF include restoration of the elbow joint anatomy with stable fixation to permit early motion.

Orthogonal Plating

The technique for orthogonal plating is the technique originally described and recommended by the AO group (**Figs. 1–8**). Patients are placed either supine with the affected extremity draped across the patients' chest or in the lateral decubitus position. A midline posterior skin incision is used with or without a slight curvature medial or lateral to the olecranon to avoid incising directly over it. It is imperative that the ulnar nerve be identified and mobilized to avoid damage to this structure. Gofton and colleagues recommended mobilizing the ulnar nerve distally to the first motor branch of the flexor carpi ulnaris. Subsequently, these investigators release the cubital tunnel retinaculum and the aponeurosis between the humeral and ulnar origins of the flexor carpi ulnaris. Proximally the intermuscular septum and Arcade of Struthers are resected. The ulnar nerve is then transposed anteriorly, with the intention to later perform a formal anterior subcutaneous transposition.[33] Other investigators feel it is unnecessary to transpose the ulnar nerve, but it does need to be mobilized enough to permit access to the distal humerus without the nerve being injured.

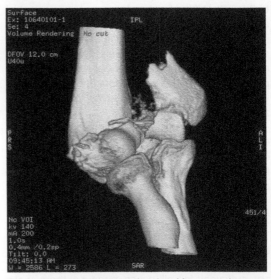

Fig. 1. Complex intraarticular distal humerus fracture. The 3-dimensional reconstruction demonstrated here can provide additional information on fracture fragment size and orientation in these complex injuries. *Courtesy of* Scott Steinmann, MD.

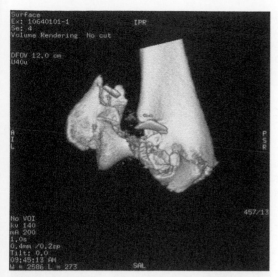

Fig. 2. Anterior 3-dimensional reconstruction of complex intraarticular distal humerus fracture subtracting the radius and ulna. Subtraction of the radius and ulna allows one to fully appreciate the fracture pattern and distinct fracture lines and articular involvement. *Courtesy of* Scott Steinmann, MD.

Once the ulnar nerve is mobilized, the distal humerus is approached through a triceps-sparing approach, a triceps-splitting approach or an olecranon osteotomy. The triceps-splitting and triceps-sparing approaches allow visualization of

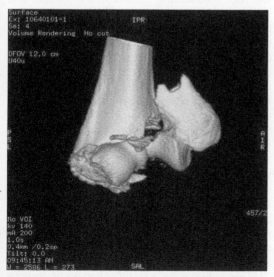

Fig. 3. Posterior 3-dimensional (3D) reconstruction of complex intraarticular distal humerus fracture subtracting the radius and ulna. The 3-D construct can be rotated in real time in many planes to allow a thorough understanding of the fracture. *Courtesy of* Scott Steinmann, MD.

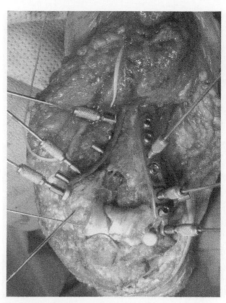

Fig. 4. Intraoperative view of ORIF of this fracture using a 90-90 plating technique. Note the placement of the plates and the preliminary K-wires, which are placed to aid in the reduction and allow easier plate application. Precontoured plates can make plate application easier, but some contouring may still be necessary. *Courtesy of* Scott Steinmann, MD.

the posterior portion of the trochlea, but only the olecranon osteotomy permits access to the anterior portions of the trochlea and capitellum.[34] The rationale for using a triceps sparing or triceps splitting approach is to avoid the complications of an olecranon osteotomy, such as prominent

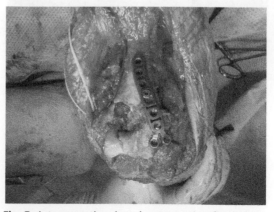

Fig. 5. Intraoperative view demonstrating final placement of the plates applied using a 90-90 plating technique. Note the excellent reduction achieved and the excellent visualization allowed using an olecranon osteotomy. *Courtesy of* Scott Steinmann, MD.

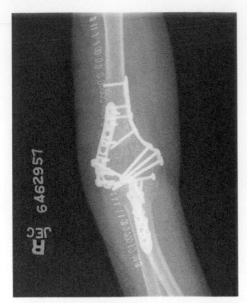

Fig. 6. Intraoperative view demonstrating final placement of the plates applied using a 90-90 plating technique. Note the excellent reduction achieved and the excellent visualization allowed using an olecranon osteotomy. *Courtesy of* Scott Steinmann, MD.

hardware, delayed unions, or nonunions. Despite these complications, the olecranon osteotomy is thought to provide optimal exposure to the intraarticular surface of the distal humerus. In addition,

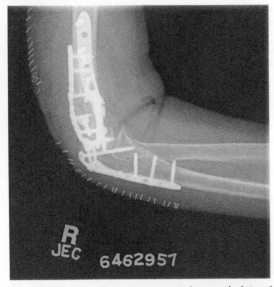

Fig. 7. Postoperative anteroposterior and lateral radiographs demonstrating anatomic reduction with union using a 90-90 plating technique. Note the fixation of the olecranon osteotomy using a precontoured olecranon plate. *Courtesy of* Scott Steinmann, MD.

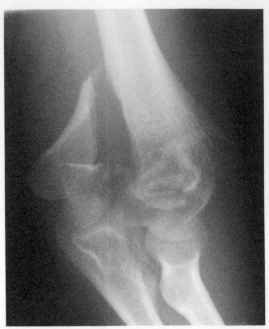

Fig. 8. Postoperative anteroposterior and lateral radiographs demonstrating anatomic reduction with union using a 90-90 plating technique. Note the fixation of the olecranon osteotomy using a precontoured olecranon plate. *Courtesy of* Scott Steinmann, MD.

by performing the osteotomy, complications involving the triceps can be avoided. These complications include disrupting the elbow extensor mechanism, fibrosis of the triceps, and intramuscular nerve injuries.[35] Mckee and colleagues[36,37] retrospectively compared patient outcomes between the triceps-splitting approach and olecranon osteotomies in a series of open distal humerus fractures and in a series of closed distal humerus fractures. Patient outcome measures, including DASH scores, the Mayo elbow score, and the 36-Item Short Form Health Survey (SF-36) scores, were recorded. The investigators of both series reported better outcomes with the triceps-splitting approach compared with an olecranon osteotomy.[36,37]

The olecranon osteotomy is started with the use of an oscillating saw but it is not completed. An osteotome is used to complete the osteotomy. If the distal humeral fracture does not have significant articular segment comminution, a triceps-splitting approach to the distal humerus can be performed. This procedure is done by reflecting equal portions of the medial and lateral triceps aponeurosis and detaching them off of the olecranon. Lastly, a triceps-sparing approach can be used with extra-articular fractures or simple intraarticular fractures by working medial and lateral to the triceps.

Once the fracture fragments are identified and reduced, provisional fixation is performed with Kirschner wires. Care must be taken here to pay attention to neurovascular structures around the elbow because the provisional Kirschner wires can injure these structures if left too long or too sharp. The orthogonal plates are then applied to the bone with the medial one being placed along the medial column of the distal humerus and the second plate being placed along the posterolateral aspect of the lateral column. The fixation should ideally have at least 3 screws proximal and 3 screws distal to the fracture site through each plate and thus through each column. When reconstruction plates are used, insufficient stability may be present and require placing a third reconstruction plate along the lateral aspect of the lateral column. This procedure was necessary in 40% of subjects in the Gofton and colleagues[33] series of AO type C distal humerus fractures.

Once the plates are secured to the distal humerus, the elbow range of motion is assessed to ensure adequate stability is present without a mechanical block. If the triceps-splitting approach was performed, the triceps are reattached to the olecranon via a nonabsorbable suture passed through drill holes in the olecranon. The medial and lateral aspects of the triceps aponeurosis are subsequently sutured to each other and the remainder of the wound is closed in layers.

If an olecranon osteotomy was performed, multiple techniques are available to provide fixation of the osteotomy site. These techniques include using a tension band, intramedullary screw fixation with or without a tension band, or placement of an olecranon plate. If an intramedullary screw is placed, it must be of sufficient size and length to obtain adequate purchase in the proximal ulna. Gofton and colleagues recommended using a contoured 3.5 mm reconstruction plate to provide the most reproducible results. Their series had no nonunions and no isolated procedures for hardware removal.[33] Additionally, the investigators stated that less morbidity is associated with hardware removal compared with reoperation for an olecranon nonunion.[33] Other investigators prefer a stronger plate, such as an limited contact dynamic compression plate, with or without locking screws to provide additional strength to the construct. Lastly, if one chooses to fix the olecranon osteotomy with a tension-band technique, an option is to use two 20-gauge wires to create two figure-of-eight tension bands. This small wire size may obviate the need for hardware removal and avoid other potential hardware-related complications.

Parallel Plating

The technique for parallel plating was described in 2007 by O'Driscoll and colleagues[23] from the Mayo Clinic (**Figs. 9–13**). Patients are positioned in the supine position and a sterile tourniquet is applied. Subsequently a triceps-anconeus reflecting pedicle (TRAP) approach is performed after the ulnar nerve is transposed anteriorly. The goal of the TRAP approach is to reflect the triceps in continuity with the anconeus. The use of an olecranon osteotomy is recommended when intra-articular comminution is present.[27]

Attention is initially directed at the articular surface of the distal humerus to ensure an adequate reduction. The articular surface is reassembled with smooth Kirschner wires to provisionally hold the reduction in place using the proximal portion of the ulna and radial head as templates if necessary. The Kirschner wires should be placed close to the subchondral bone to ensure that they do not interfere with placement of your screws into the distal fragment. If during the reduction missing bone is encountered, one should understand that the anterior aspect of the distal part of the humerus is the critical area that needs to be restored to allow for a functional joint.[27] The posterior aspect of the articular surface of the distal humerus is a less critical region. In addition, the medial half of the trochlea is vital to ensure stability of the elbow articulation. It can be reconstructed with either the lateral half of the trochlea or the capitellum.[27]

Once the articular surface is anatomically reduced, the plates are placed along the medial and lateral columns of the distal humerus. One-third tubular plates are not strong enough for fixation of these fractures and therefore the

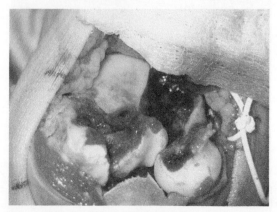

Fig. 9. Preoperative anteroposterior and lateral radiographs demonstrating a complex intraarticular fracture of the distal humerus. *Courtesy of* David Ring, MD.

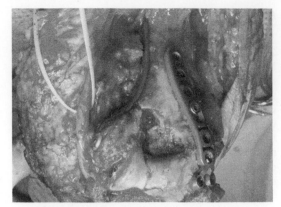

Fig. 10. Preoperative anteroposterior and lateral radiographs demonstrating a complex intraarticular fracture of the distal humerus. *Courtesy of* David Ring, MD.

precontoured distal humerus plates are currently favored. However, if the surgeon is contouring the plates, it should be recognized that it is preferable to undercontour the plates to allow for additional compression at the metaphyseal region when they are applied. The plates should be long enough to allow for at least 3 screws to be placed in the proximal part of the humeral shaft proximal to the metaphyseal component of the fracture. Additionally, the plates should end at different levels to avoid creating a stress riser.[27]

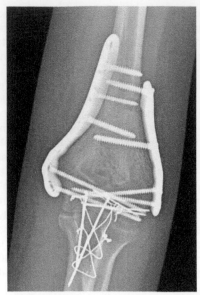

Fig. 12. Postoperative anteroposterior and lateral radiographs demonstrating anatomic reduction and union of this complex distal humerus fracture using a parallel-plating technique. Note the number of screws that can be placed in the distal fragments. In addition, the olecranon osteotomy has been fixed using a double-wire tension-band technique. *Courtesy of* David Ring, MD.

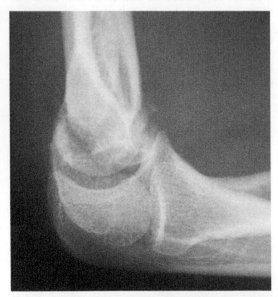

Fig. 11. Intraoperative view of this complex distal humerus fracture. The vessel loop is protecting the ulnar nerve, which should be mobilized routinely in all of these complex cases. An olecranon osteotomy has been performed to aid in fracture visualization. *Courtesy of* David Ring, MD.

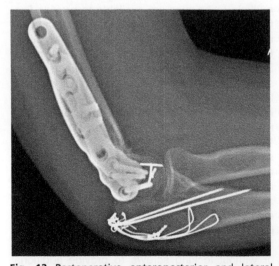

Fig. 13. Postoperative anteroposterior and lateral radiographs demonstrating anatomic reduction and union of this complex distal humerus fracture using a parallel-plating technique. Note the number of screws that can be placed in the distal fragments. In addition, the olecranon osteotomy has been fixed using a double-wire tension-band technique. *Courtesy of* David Ring, MD.

Once the appropriate size plates are chosen, they are held in place by driving a smooth Steinmann pin through the respective epicondyle, medially or laterally. Subsequently, 1 cortical screw is introduced in the slotted hole of each plate to accommodate for minor adjustments in plate position. Following adjustment of plate height, a large bone clamp is used to compress the intraarticular fracture fragments, supposing there is no missing bone. This procedure allows for interfragmentary compression of the intraarticular fragments without the need for lag screws. Once the clamp is in place, the distal screws are inserted to secure the intraarticular fragments to the plates. These distal screws should be as long as possible, pass through as many fragments as possible, and engage the opposite column.[27]

Once the distal fragments are secured to the plates, attention is turned to the supracondylar region. One of the screws in the slotted holes is backed out and a large bone clamp is placed to eccentrically load the supracondylar region. This procedure is accomplished by placing the clamp distally on the side the screw was backed out of and proximally on the opposite side. A proximal screw is then inserted in compression mode and the slotted screw is retightened.[27] During this maneuver it is important to ensure that the varus-valgus and rotational alignments were not altered. The same process of loosening the slotted screw, applying the bone clamp, placing a proximal screw, and retightening the slotted screw is now performed on the opposite side. The remaining screws are now placed to allow for additional stability. The holes created by the Steinmann pins in the epicondyles can be used as pilot holes for placement of screws into these areas.[27]

Once the plates are affixed to the humerus, the elbow is taken through a range of motion of flexion-extension and pronation-supination to ensure no mechanical blocks are present. One deep and one subcutaneous drain are placed and the wounds are closed. The arm is then placed in a bulky noncompressive dressing with an anterior plaster splint to maintain full extension. The dressing is removed approximately 3 to 5 days postoperatively and physical therapy, including active and passive motion, is begun.

OUTCOMES
Orthogonal Plating

Gofton and colleagues performed a retrospective review of 23 subjects treated with dual orthogonal plates at a mean follow-up of 45 months. Their results demonstrated that subjects had minimal subjective deficits (10%) with a mean overall satisfaction score of 93%. The mean DASH (Disabilities of the Arm, Shoulder, and Hand) score at the most recent follow-up was 12, with a range from 0 to 38; whereas the mean ASES (American Shoulder and Elbow Surgeons) score was 9.7, plus or minus 10.1 points. The mean amount of flexion achieved was 142° with a mean flexion contracture of 19°. No significant differences in pronation or supination were noted between the affected and unaffected sides. A statistically significant decrease in strength was present in all strength parameters assessed.[33]

Assessment of the postoperative radiographs did not demonstrate any distal humeral articular step-offs or gaps greater than 2 mm. In addition, there were no nonunions or malunions indentified in the distal humerus. The amount of posttraumatic arthritis present, as classified by Knirk and Jupiter, was grade 0 or 1 in 18 subjects, and grade 2 or 3 in 5 subjects.[33,38]

Parallel Plating

Sanchez-Sotelo and colleagues discussed their retrospective results of 32 subjects treated with parallel plating over a 10-year period when they described the surgical technique. Thirty-one of the 32 subjects went on to union without requiring additional surgery and none of the subjects had failure of their hardware or fracture displacement.[23] The average flexion-extension arc at the latest follow-up was 99° but 5 subjects did require excision of heterotopic ossification secondary to elbow stiffness. The mean Mayo Elbow Performance Score (MEPS) was 85 points with 27 subjects having a good or excellent result and 5 subjects having a fair or poor result.[23]

Athwal and colleagues also recently published a retrospective review of AO/OTA type C fractures treated with the Mayo Elbow parallel plating system. In their series of 32 subjects, the average flexion-extension arc, at a mean of 27-months follow-up, was 97°. The mean DASH score was 24 points, whereas the mean MEPS was 82 points. They noted no implant failures and nonunions.[39]

COMPLICATIONS

Complications arise whether using the orthogonal plating technique or the parallel plating technique. These complications include heterotopic ossification, failure of fixation, nonunion, malunion, infection, ulnar neuropathy, and complex regional pain syndrome.

In the orthogonal plating series of 23 subjects by Gofton and colleagues, about half of the subjects experienced at least one complication, with the presence of heterotopic ossification being the most common (present in 30% of subjects). These investigators reported no loss of fixation and no cases of ulnar neuropathy. An olecranon nonunion was present in 2 subjects, both of which required an additional procedure to achieve union. No distal humeral nonunions or malunions were noted.[33]

In the recently published retrospective series of Athwal and colleagues assessing the Mayo Elbow parallel plate technique, they noted a complication rate of 53%, with complications arising in 17 of 32 subjects. The most common complication noted was postoperative nerve injuries, present in 5 subjects (16%) of which 3 had completely resolved by 4.5 months postoperatively. Four subjects (12%) did experience wound complications, including 2 wound dehiscences requiring surgical debridement. One olecranon nonunion was noted, which was treated nonoperatively.[39]

NONUNION SCENARIOS

Similar to the difficulties encountered treating distal humerus fractures, treatment of distal humeral nonunions has proven to be a difficult entity for the surgeon. This complication is especially devastating when elbow instability is so severe that the limb cannot be supported against gravity. Treatment of this problem can be achieved with total elbow arthroplasty, however many patients are too young or active for total elbow arthroplasty to be the optimal treatment. Therefore, some investigators have suggested using multiple plates to provide adequate stability to achieve osseous union.[26]

Ring and colleagues retrospectively reviewed 15 subjects with distal humeral nonunions treated with multiple plates to achieve adequate osseous stability. The orthogonal-plating technique, with autogenous bone-grafting, was performed in 5 subjects, whereas the remaining subjects required a third or fourth plate to achieve adequate fixation. Twelve of the 15 subjects achieved union, whereas the remaining 3 subjects went on to have a total elbow arthroplasty performed. After a minimum of a 2-year follow-up, the average flexion achieved was 117° with a flexion contracture present averaging 22°. Eleven of the 12 subjects who achieved union had excellent or good functional results according to the MEPS.[40]

SUMMARY

Distal humerus fractures continue to be a complex fracture for the surgeon to treat. This article describes two techniques that can be used to tackle these difficult fractures. Both of these techniques have yielded excellent outcomes after

ORIF; however, both techniques have significant complications associated with them. Use of parallel plating or orthogonal plating will depend on surgeon preference and the fracture pattern present. Orthogonal plating may be preferred in cases of an anterior shear fracture where the fixation from posterior to anterior will provide additional stability to the intraarticular fractures. Parallel plating may be the preferred technique used for very distal fracture patterns, because more stability can be obtained by providing additional screws in the distal fragment. The key to successful treatment of these fractures is obtaining anatomic reduction with stable fixation to allow early range of motion. Performing anatomic reductions while minimizing soft-tissue trauma will lead to improved patient outcomes while minimizing the complication rates.

REFERENCES

1. Srinivasan K, Agarwal M, Matthews SJE, et al. Fractures of the distal humerus in the elderly. Clin Orthop Relat Res 2005;434:222–30.
2. Robinson CM, Hill RMF, Jacobs N, et al. Adult distal humerus metaphyseal fractures: epidemiology and results of treatment. J Orthop Trauma 2003;17:38–47.
3. Muller ME, Allgower M, Schneider R, et al. Manual of internal fixation techniques recommended by the AO group. 2nd edition. New York: Springer; 1979. 176–7.
4. Jupiter JB, Mehne DK. Fractures of the distal humerus. Orthopedics 1992;15:825–33.
5. Davies MB, Stanley D. A clinically applicable fracture classification for distal humeral fractures. J Shoulder Elbow Surg 2006;15:602–8.
6. Leugmair M, Timofiev E, Chirpaz-Cerbat JM. Surgical treatment of AO type C distal humerus fractures: internal fixation with a Y-shaped reconstruction (Lambda) plate. J Shoulder Elbow Surg 2008; 17:113–20.
7. Seth AK, Baratz ME. Fractures of the elbow. In: Trumble TE, Budoff JE, Cornwall R, editors. Hand, elbow, shoulder. Philadelphia: Mosby; 2006. p. 522–31.
8. London JT. Kinematics of the elbow. J Bone Joint Surg 1981;63:529–36.
9. Mehne DK, Matta J. Bicolumn fractures of the adult humerus. In: Paper presented at the 53rd annual meeting of the American Academy of Orthopaedic Surgeons, New Orleans (LA); February, 1986.
10. McKee MD, Jupiter JB. Fractures of the distal humerus. Skeletal trauma basic science, management, and reconstruction. 3rd edition. Philadelphia: Saunders; 2003. p. 1436–80.
11. Milch H. Fractures and fracture-dislocations of the humeral condyles. J Trauma 1964;4:592–607.

12. Wickstrom J, Meyer PR. Fractures of the distal humerus in adults. Clin Orthop 1967;50:43–51.

13. Bryan RS, Morrey BF. Fractures of the distal humerus. In: Morrey BF, editor. The elbow and its disorders. Philadelphia: W.B. Saunders; 1985. p. 302–39.

14. Jupiter JB, Neff U, Holzach P, et al. Intercondylar fracture of the humerus. J Bone Joint Surg 1985; 67:226–39.

15. McKee MD, Jupiter JB. A contemporary approach to the management of complex fractures of the distal humerus and their sequelae. Hand Clin 1994;10: 479–94.

16. McKee MD, Jupiter JB, Toh CL, et al. Reconstruction after malunion and nonunion of intraarticular fractures of the distal humerus. Methods and results in 13 adults. J Bone Joint Surg Br 1994;76:614–21.

17. Waddell JP, Hatch J, Richards RR. Supracondylar fractures of the humerus: results of surgical treatment. J Trauma 1988;28:1615–21.

18. Henley MB, Bone LB, Parker B. Operative management of intra-articular fractures of the distal humerus. J Orthop Trauma 1987;1:24–35.

19. Letsch R, Schmit-Neuerburg KP, Sturmer KM, et al. Intraarticular fractures of the distal humerus. Surgical treatment and results. Clin Orthop Relat Res 1989;241:238–44.

20. Holdsworth BJ, Mossad MM. Fractures of the adult distal humerus. Elbow function after internal fixation. J Bone Joint Surg Br 1990;72:362–5.

21. Wildburger R, Mahring M, Hofer HP. Supraintercondylar fractures of the distal humerus: results of internal fixation. J Orthop Trauma 1991;5:301–7.

22. Sodegard J, Sandelin J, Bostman O. Postoperative complications of distal humeral fractures. 27/96 adults followed up for 6 (2–10) years. Acta Orthop Scand 1992;63:85–9.

23. Sanchez-Sotelo J, Torchia ME, O'Driscoll SW. Complex distal humeral fractures: Internal fixation with a principle-based parallel-plate technique. J Bone Joint Surg Am 2007;89:961–9.

24. Ackerman G, Jupiter JB. Non-union of fractures of the distal end of the humerus. J Bone Joint Surg Am 1988;70:75–83.

25. Korner J, Diederichs G, Arzdorf M, et al. A biomechanical evaluation of methods of distal humerus fracture fixation using locking compression plates versus conventional reconstruction plates. J Orthop Trauma 2004;18:286–93.

26. Ring D, Jupiter JB. Fractures of the distal humerus. Orthop Clin North Am 2000;31:103–13.

27. Sanchez-Sotelo J, Torchia ME, O'Driscoll SW. Complex distal humeral fractures: Internal fixation with a principle-based parallel-plate technique. Surgical technique. J Bone Joint Surg Am 2008; 90(Suppl 2):31–46.

28. Self J, Viegas SF Jr, Buford WL, et al. A comparison of double-plate fixation methods for complex distal humerus fractures. J Shoulder Elbow Surg 1995;4: 10–6.

29. Jacobson SR, Glisson RR, Urbanaik JR. Comparison of distal humerus fracture fixation: a biomechanical study. J South Orthop Assoc 1997;6:241–9.

30. Schwartz A, Oka R, Odell T, et al. Biomechanical comparison of two perpendicular plating systems for stabilization of complex distal humerus fractures. Clin Biomech (Bristol, Avon) 2006;21:950–5.

31. Stoffel K, Cunnenn S, Morgan R, et al. Comparative stability of perpendicular versus parallel double-locking plating systems in osteoporotic comminuted distal humerus fractures. J Orthop Res 2008;26:778–84.

32. Schuster I, Korner J, Arzdorf M, et al. Mechanical comparison in cadaver specimens of three different 90-degree double-plate osteosyntheses for simulated C2-type distal humerus fractures with varying bone densities. J Orthop Trauma 2008;22:113–20.

33. Gofton WT, MacDermid JC, Patterson SD, et al. Functional outcome of AO type C distal humeral fractures. J Hand Surg Am 2003;28:294–308.

34. Wong AS, Baratz ME. Elbow fractures: distal humerus. J Hand Surg Am 2009;34:176–90.

35. Bryan RS, Morrey BF. Extensive posterior exposure of the elbow. A triceps-sparing approach. Clin Orthop 1982;166:188–92.

36. McKee MD, Wilson TL, Winston L, et al. Functional outcome following surgical treatment of intra-articular distal humeral fractures through a posterior approach. J Bone Joint Surg Am 2000;82:1701–7.

37. McKee MD, Kim J, Kebaish K, et al. Functional outcome after open supracondylar fractures of the huemrus. The effect of the surgical approach. J Bone Joint Surg Br 2000;82:646–51.

38. Knirk JL, Jupiter JB. Intraarticular fractures of the distal end of the radius in young adults. J Bone Joint Surg Am 1986;68:647–59.

39. Athwal GS, Hoxie SC, Rispoli DM, et al. Precontoured parallel plate fixation of AO/OTA type C distal humerus fractures. J Orthop Trauma 2009;23:575–80.

40. Ring D, Gulotta L, Jupiter JB. Unstable nonunions of the distal part of the humerus. J Bone Joint Surg Am 2003;85:1040–6.

Hinged External Fixation of the Elbow

Neal C. Chen, MD[a],*, Abhishek Julka, MD[b]

KEYWORDS

• External fixation • Elbow • Hinge • Instability

External fixation is a method of semi-rigid immobilization with fixation exclusive of the injury zone. First described in the use of patellar fractures, external fixators have evolved substantially in their composition and versatility. Static fixators have been used in the traumatic setting across various joints. However, static external fixation is problematic in the elbow. In particular, prolonged immobilization can lead to loss of motion and pain.[1]

Hinged external fixation provides advantages of static fixation while permitting joint range of motion. In the elbow, hinged external fixation can be used for several specific purposes: (1) maintaining a stable, congruent ulnohumeral joint; (2) allowing acutely injured soft tissues to heal relative to the axis of the hinged fixator; (3) allowing chronically injured soft tissue to contract relative to the axis of the hinged fixator; and (4) distracting the joint while maintaining axis of rotation.

Hinged external fixation has been used in the setting of traumatic instability, distraction interposition arthroplasty (DIA), and contracture release. Each of these applications requires an understanding of goals and pitfalls of hinged external fixation.

BIOMECHANICS

The elbow joint is formed by the articulation of the distal humerus, proximal ulna, and proximal radius. The angle formed by the anatomic axis of the humerus and ulna in the plane of the humerus with the elbow in extension is referred to as the carrying angle. This angle is approximately 10° to 15° in men and 15° to 17° in women.[2] Motion

about the elbow joint is described by flexion-extension and pronation-supination. Flexion-extension occurs at the ulnohumeral articulation, whereas pronation-supination occurs through the forearm with the radius rotating about the ulna. Most activities of daily living require elbow range of motion of 30° to 130° flexion-extension and 50° each of pronation and supination.[3]

The flexion-extension axis of the elbow is of particular importance to hinged external fixation. Ideally, the axis of the hinged external fixator should be coincident with the axis of rotation at all degrees of elbow flexion. Studies of the instant center of rotation have described an area 2 to 3 mm in diameter located at the center of the trochlea through which the instant center of rotation passes. Qualitatively, the axis of rotation passes through the center of the arcs formed by the trochlear sulcus and capitellum. The axis is internally rotated 3° to 8° in respect to the plane of the epicondyles, and forms an angle of 82° to 86° with the axis of the humerus (**Fig. 1**). The anatomic landmarks for locating the axis of rotation are the tubercle of the origin of the lateral collateral ligament and anterior and inferior to the medial epicondyle.[3] Precise replication of the axis is important, because 5 mm of translation or 5° of angulation results in a fourfold increase in resistance to flexion.[4]

PRINCIPLES OF EXTERNAL FIXATION

At the most basic level, a hinged external fixator consists of two rigid bodies whose motion relative to one another is constrained to a fixed axis.

[a] Medsport, Department of Orthopaedic Surgery, University of Michigan, 24 Frank Lloyd Wright Drive Lobby A, Ann Arbor, MI 48106-0391, USA
[b] Department of Orthopaedic Surgery, University of Michigan, 1500 E. Medical Center Drive, 2912 Taubman Center, Ann Arbor, MI 48109-5328, USA
* Corresponding author.
E-mail address: chenneal@med.umich.edu

Hand Clin 26 (2010) 423–433
doi:10.1016/j.hcl.2010.04.004

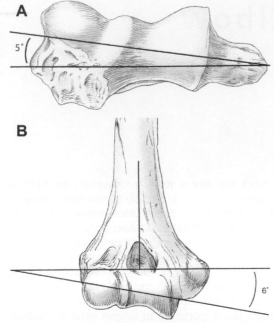

Fig. 1. (*A*) Axis of the elbow is internally rotated 3° to 8° relative to the epicondylar axis. (*B*) Axis of the elbow lies approximately 82° to 86° valgus relative to the axis of the humerus (4° to 8° relative to the perpendicular to the axis). *From* Morrey BF. Chapter 2. Anatomy of the elbow joint. In: Morrey BF, editor. The elbow and its disorders. Elsevier; 2009. p. 18; with permission.

Hinged external fixation of the elbow involves ensuring that the axis of rotation of the two rigid bodies is coincident with the axis of rotation of the elbow, and rigidly securing the humerus to one body and the ulna to the other body.

An external fixator neutralizes forces across the injured segment until enough healing has occurred such that the elbow can accept those forces. At the same time, a hinged external fixator allows motion through the elbow joint to allow the soft tissues to heal with proper gliding planes and approximately correct length and tension.

From a practical standpoint, external fixators provide structural support to an injured extremity with fixation outside of the zone of injury. In the same manner, a fixator can also serve as an adjunct to internal fixation. External fixators allow access to the area of injury for secondary procedures and allow for manipulation of injured segments through the fixator.

The basic structural component of an external fixator is pins fixed to the bone with interconnecting rigid bars. These structural components provide some degree of inherent rigidity. In addition, the stiffness of the frame can be improved by increasing pin diameter, pin-to-pin distance,

reducing rod-to-bone distance, multiplanar application, stacking bars, and the use of thicker or more rigid components.[5,6]

Hinged fixators share structural and biomechanical properties with static fixators, with the additional advantage of allowing movement in one or more planes. This additional mobility alters the ability of a hinged fixator to control the fracture. Multiple investigators have studied the biomechanics of the hinged external fixator. Kamineni and colleagues[7] investigated the varus/valgus and forearm rotational displacements associated with collateral ligament injuries with application of a laterally based hinged external fixator. In the presence of medial and lateral collateral ligament injuries, they found that valgus stability is lost with addition of any load. Kamineni and colleagues concluded that medial soft tissue injury may be incompletely controlled with unilateral fixators. A separate cadaveric study demonstrated stiffness in varus to be 4 times that in valgus.[8] The decreased ability of a uniplanar fixator to control valgus laxity should be considered and the instability pattern assessed carefully before choosing a particular fixator.

Distraction of the joint surface is a feature available in most hinged external fixators. Distraction functions to neutralize contact forces across the joint, allows for immediate postoperative motion, and prevents ligamentous healing in a contracted position. Sekiya and colleagues[8] performed a cadaveric study with a uniplanar lateral fixator axially loading the elbow with varying degrees of joint contact. These investigators determined distraction to decrease the overall stiffness of the system. Although distraction is used in few applications it is important to consider this problem, especially with interposition arthroplasty, where distraction is used but ulnohumeral instability is a problem.

FIXATOR APPLICATION

Although fixator application varies from manufacturer to manufacturer, they have some shared surgical principles. The procedure requires precise radiographic determination of the ulnohumeral axis of rotation. The ulnohumeral axis passes between the lateral epicondyle and inferior to the medial epicondyle. The axis pin should pass parallel to the trochlea on the anteroposterior (AP) view and pass through the center of the trochlea on the lateral view (**Fig. 2**).

An axis pin may be placed at this point. Technique points for placing the axis pin are: (1) place a towel over the receiver to protect it from the axis pin; (2) obtain a precise lateral fluoroscopic image; (3) identify the starting point with the axis

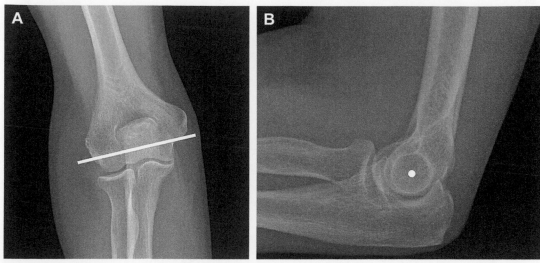

Fig. 2. (*A*) AP radiograph of the elbow. The line indicates the axis of the ulnohumeral joint. (*B*) Lateral radiograph of the elbow. The dot indicates the axis of the ulnohumeral joint.

pin; and (4) on securing the starting point, rotate the pin such that it is perfectly colinear with the radiographic source.

The hinge is placed over the axis pin. From there, the humeral and ulnar aspects of the fixator are applied with standard external fixation techniques. Care should be taken in placing the proximal humeral pin, because the radial nerve is in close proximity. If a multiplanar fixator is applied, the ulnar nerve is transposed subcutaneously and the medial pin placed.

FIXATOR TYPES

Hinged elbow external fixators are categorized as uniplanar or multiplanar. A uniplanar hinged fixator consists of a simple articulation that allows flexion and extension, but constrains valgus/varus and rotation relative to that fixed axis. A multiplanar fixator offers control of the elbow in multiple planes and consists of an articulation that allows flexion-extension. The multiplanar fixator ultimately offers more control of the axis of rotation. Unilateral fixators are lower profile and technically easier to apply, whereas multiplanar fixator offers increased stability at the consequence of greater technical difficulty and bulkier design.

Several hinged elbow external fixators are currently available. Although there are differences between them, each shares certain common structural principles. These fixators provide a stable frame to which the humerus and ulna are attached, a hinge that is coaxial with the ulnohumeral joint, the ability for the elbow to move actively, and the potential to distract the joint relative to the axis of the ulnohumeral joint.

Of the commercially available uniplanar fixators, 3 have been in use for several years. The Dynamic Joint Distractor II (DJD II) (Stryker Howmedica Osteonics, Mahwah, NJ) is a low-profile unilateral fixator with the advantage of unilateral or bilateral application (**Fig. 3**). The DJD II is a kit that allows the Hoffman II Compact external fixation system to be applied to the elbow. It is simple in design, such that once the axis pin is placed, the hinge can be slid on the axis pin and the remainder of the fixator can be constructed relative to the hinge. In a similar manner, the Synthes Arm hinge (Synthes, Paoli, PA) couples with the Synthes large external fixator to expand the capabilities of the basic fixator set (**Fig. 4**). If additional stability is needed, a fixator may also be applied to the medial side.

The Orthofix (Intavent Orthofix Ltd, Berkshire, UK) elbow fixator is a unilateral frame fixator. The primary advantage of the Orthofix fixator is that there are fewer modular elements than in those hinge systems that are extensions of a basic external fixation kit. The fixator elements allow for a large degree of rotation and angulation to allow pin placement. One disadvantage with this system is that there is a specific order of locking the fixator elements, and failure to follow this order may result in improper hinge function.

The OptiROM (Biomet EBI, Parsippany, NJ, USA) elbow fixator is a unilateral fixator that can be placed radiographically to avoid using a pin to localize the axis of rotation (**Fig. 5**). Radiographic placement is useful when suture anchors, screws, or other hardware may interfere with axis pin placement. This benefit is particularly useful in the setting of acute trauma where the elbow is

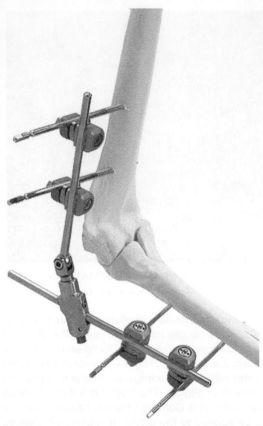

Fig. 3. DJD II. *Courtesy of* Stryker Howmedica Osteonics, Mahwah, NJ. Used with permission.

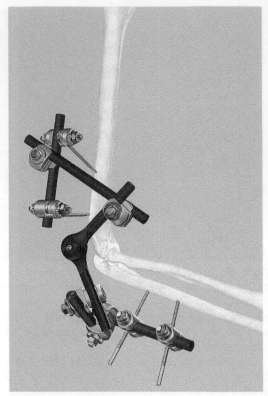

Fig. 4. Synthes Arm. *Images courtesy of* Synthes Inc., West Chester, PA; with permission. © 2009 Synthes, Inc., or its affiliates.

found to be unstable in retrospect after fixation has been placed. Unlike axis pin guidance, radiographic placement involves securing the fixator to the humerus, aligning the targeting guide and then securing the ulna relative to the targeting guide/fixator.

The Compass hinge (Smith & Nephew, Memphis, TN, USA) is a multiplanar external fixator (**Fig. 6**). This fixator is more versatile, but is also a more technically demanding fixator to apply than a uniplanar fixator. Advantages of this fixator include: (1) a radiolucent frame; (2) adjustment of varus-valgus of the axis of rotation; and (3) a gear mechanism that allows passive range of motion. Disadvantages include the bulk of the frame and a higher potential of developing skin problems because of impingement on the fixed frame secondary to swelling.

ACUTE INSTABILITY

Acute elbow instability includes a large variety of pathologic entities, ranging from simple elbow dislocation to complex fracture dislocations of the elbow. Simple elbow dislocations are generally stable after reduction and a short course of immobilization. However, there is the rare occurrence when a simple dislocation requires additional surgical intervention. Dislocations with associated fracture disturbing the osseous restraints of the elbow may require external fixation to maintain stable fracture reduction and allow postoperative motion. The hinged external fixator has been used for acute injury in the setting of severe simple instability or acute complex instability.

Figs. 7–11 demonstrate a case of a capitellar/lateral column fracture sustained by a 60-year-old woman who fell onto her elbow. She was placed in a splint for a week before presentation at the authors' institution. Radiographs demonstrated persistent dislocation despite closed reduction in the emergency department (see **Figs. 7** and **8**). The soft tissues were blistered and it was believed that the swelling prohibited operative intervention at that time. A static fixator was placed to reduce the ulnohumeral joint and to allow the edema to subside (see **Fig. 9**). After 10 days, the skin condition had improved to allow for an operative intervention. Open reduction and internal fixation were performed. The lateral column was impacted from the prolonged initial dislocation; so a bone

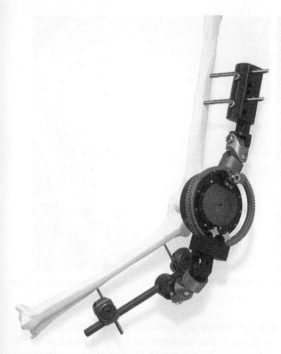

Fig. 5. Optirom. *Courtesy of* Biomet EBI, Parsippany, NJ. Used with permission; copyright © 2009 Biomet Trauma.

graft substitute was added to supplement the lateral column. Because the fixation was tenuous, a hinged external fixator was added to protect the internal construct and to maintain joint congruity (see **Fig. 10**). Once the bone had healed sufficiently, the external fixator was removed (see **Fig. 11**). Range of motion at 3 months postoperatively was 30° to 110° of flexion-extension and 70° each of pronation and supination.

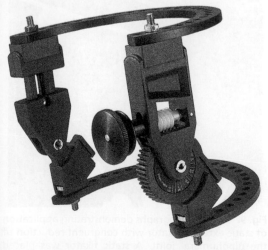

Fig. 6. Compass hinge. *Courtesy of* Smith & Nephew, Memphis, TN; with permission.

Hinged external fixation maintains concentric reduction of the ulnohumeral joint while minimizing external forces on the soft tissues and osseous structures about the elbow. The most common situation in which an external fixator is used for acute instability is with a fracture dislocation of the elbow whereby internal fixation is insufficient to maintain osseous stability with early motion. In this application, hinged external fixation decreases the forces experienced by the fracture-hardware construct to minimize displacement.

Stavlas and colleagues[9] have used a unilateral hinged external fixator in fracture dislocations of severely osteoporotic elbows after the internal fixation was deemed insufficient in a small cohort of patients, with good results. Application of a hinged external fixator may also be performed in the perioperative period. Ruch and Triepel[10] describe a cohort of 8 patients who failed to maintain concentric reduction following open reduction and internal fixation for fracture dislocation of the elbow. A subgroup of patients was treated with a hinged external fixator within 6 weeks of the index procedure. This subgroup maintained concentric reduction after hinged fixator placement and had functional range of motion after fixator removal. McKee and colleagues[11] also describe treatment of a cohort of patients with acute recurrent instability after open reduction and internal fixation using a hinged fixator, with similar results. Yu and colleagues[12] demonstrated the use of a multiplanar fixator in recurrent elbow dislocation with and without associated fractures. A large majority of the patients obtained a concentrically reduced joint with functional range of motion.

Duckworth and colleagues[13] describe the rare phenomenon of ulnohumeral instability without fracture requiring operative intervention. In these cases, a reasonable approach is to repair the collateral ligaments, and if there is persistent instability, a hinged fixator may be applied. The investigators also describe cross-pinning the ulnohumeral joint in situations where there are extenuating circumstances. Hinged external fixation is used in this situation to maintain concentric reduction of the ulnohumeral joint until the soft tissues have healed enough to prevent joint subluxation or dislocation under physiologic loads. Although operative intervention for elbow dislocation is usually unnecessary, knowledge of these salvage techniques is important.

CHRONIC INSTABILITY

The spectrum of chronic instability ranges from occasional subluxation to locked dislocation. Like acute elbow instability, these cases may

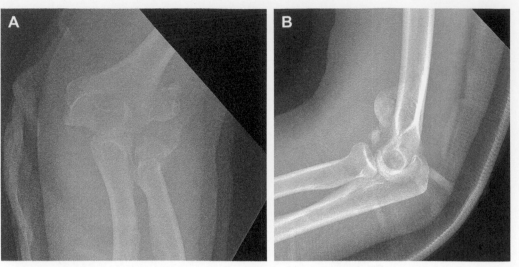

Fig. 7. (*A*) AP and (*B*) lateral radiographs of an unreduced capitellar fracture/lateral column fracture that had occurred 1 week before presentation.

have accompanying fractures of the proximal ulna and radius and the distal humerus. Much attention has been paid to simple, recurrent elbow instability treated with lateral ulnar collateral ligament reconstruction. However, for those unstable elbows with either malunited or ununited fractures or elbows that have been persistently dislocated, hinged external fixation has been a successful treatment modality. In the case of chronic instability, the goal of the hinged external fixation is to provide a reference axis to which the soft tissues heal and contract. Unlike acute injury, where there is

enough tissue disruption to affect a robust healing response, the success of hinged fixation in the setting of chronic instability is not as predictable.

In the previously mentioned study by Ruch and Triepel,[10] a subgroup of patients had a subluxed ulnohumeral joint more than 6 weeks after initial open reduction and internal fixation. These patients were treated with placement of a hinged

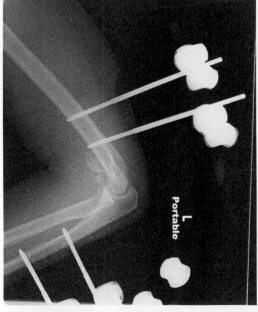

Fig. 9. Lateral radiographs demonstrating application of static external fixator with congruent reduction of the ulnohumeral joint. A static fixator was placed because of the presence of fracture blisters that precluded definitive fixation.

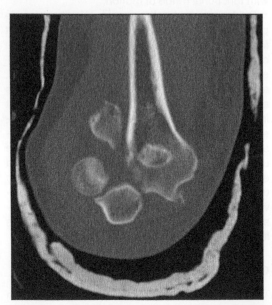

Fig. 8. Computed tomography demonstrating capitellar fragment and lateral column insufficiency.

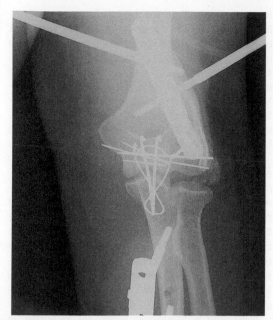

Fig. 10. Radiographs demonstrating internal fixation of the capitellar fragment with threaded k-wires, posterior capitellar plate (Synthes, Paoli, PA, USA), bone graft, and application Compass Hinged External Fixator (Smith & Nephew, Memphis, TN, USA) with reduction of the ulnohumeral joint.

external fixator and were maintained reduction at the time of final follow-up; however, most of them did not regain functional range of motion. The outcomes of hinged fixator application for late traumatic instability do not seem as robust as those for acute traumatic instability.

Jupiter and Ring[14] treated 5 patients with chronically unreduced elbow dislocations without

associated fractures. The patients underwent: (1) open debridement of granulation tissue that had been deposited in the joint; (2) reduction; (3) re-approximation of soft tissues en bloc to the lateral epicondyle; and (4) application of Compass external fixator placement. Passive motion with the use of the gear mechanism was started immediately, with active motion beginning 10 to 14 days postoperatively. At an average follow-up of 38 months, all patients demonstrated stable, concentrically reduced joints. Patients regained full supination-pronation, but had a flexion contracture of about 15°.

DISTRACTION INTERPOSITION ARTHROPLASTY

There is no durable, consistent surgical solution for elbow arthritis in the young, active individual. Semi-constrained arthroplasty has been used with limited success, although it requires the individual to modulate their functional activities. Distraction arthroplasty and interposition arthroplasty without distraction have also been attempted historically, with mixed results. DIA is the confluence of these two techniques to (1) gain the advantages of distraction to protect the interposition in the subacute postoperative period and (2) limit instability postoperatively. Results from these techniques demonstrate some improvements from distraction or interposition alone, but outcomes remain guarded. Pain relief is unpredictable and postoperative instability remains a problem.

The procedure involves dislocation of the ulnohumeral joint without takedown of the triceps

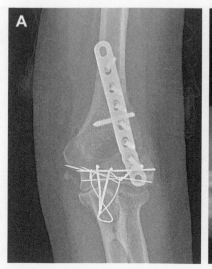
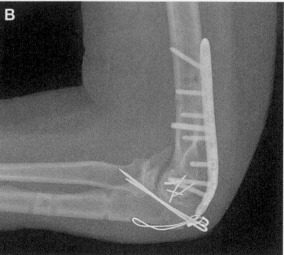

Fig. 11. (*A*) AP and (*B*) lateral radiographs demonstrating maintenance of ulnohumeral congruence after removal of fixator.

mechanism.[15] The lateral collateral ligaments and the common extensor origins are released from the humerus and, if necessary, the medial ulnar collateral ligament and the common flexor origin.[16] The distal humerus and ulnohumeral joint are prepared to accept the interposition material. The radial head is resected if it blocks forearm rotation. Cheng and Morrey[17] describe a radialization procedure in some instances by resecting the ulnar articular margin for the radial head to aid forearm rotation. The graft is laid over the distal humerus articular surface and held in place with sutures placed through drill holes or suture anchors. The collateral ligaments are reattached and hinged external fixator applied with 3 to 4 mm of distraction. Early motion is initiated and the fixator is removed after a minimum of 3 weeks.

Cheng and Morrey[17] have reported on 13 patients with painful, mobile, arthritic elbows treated with DIA, using fascia lata autograft and the Dynamic Joint Distractor (Stryker Howmedica Osteonics, Mahwah, NJ, USA). The primary indication for surgery in these cases was pain. The Mayo elbow performance score showed 4 excellent, 4 good, 1 fair, and 4 poor results, with 9 patients having improvement in pain. Four patients eventually required total elbow arthroplasty. All patients with instability following the procedure had unsatisfactory results.

Nolla and colleagues[16] retrospectively reviewed 13 patients with stiff, posttraumatic elbow arthrosis. The indication for surgery in these patients was limited range of motion in addition to pain. DIA with an Achilles allograft was performed with a Compass hinge fixator (Smith & Nephew, Memphis, TN, USA). The fixator was removed at an average of 7 weeks. Eleven patients who maintained the DIA at 4 years demonstrated a 41-point average improvement in the Broberg-Morrey score. Of the 7 patients who returned for follow-up examination, 1 rated the elbow as excellent, 5 good, and 1 fair. However, 4 of the patients had severe instability postoperatively.

From these studies, the response of hinged external fixation may be more akin to the treatment of chronic instability rather than the treatment of acute instability. In these cases of posttraumatic arthrosis, although the elbow may be stiff, the bony constraints limiting the range of motion may hide underlying ligamentous instability.[16] Despite the acute trauma of the operation, there is likely attenuation of the collateral ligaments that respond more like chronically injured tissue.

A second confounding factor for instability in these cases is the use of distraction. Although the 3 to 4 mm of distraction is intended to compensate for the bone loss during preparation of the joint surfaces, it is also possible that distraction of the soft tissues during the course of several weeks may contribute to ligament attenuation and postoperative instability.

Finally, in these small series it is difficult to determine whether postoperative instability is related to soft-tissue attenuation or to the loss of bony geometry. In the latter case, once the hinged external fixator is removed, if the bony

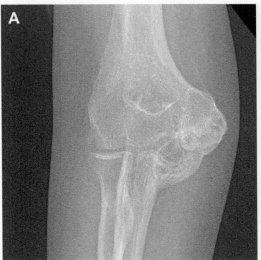
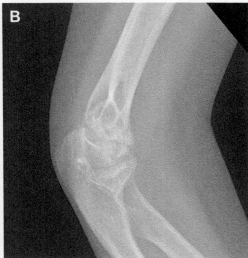

Fig. 12. (*A*) AP and (*B*) Lateral radiographs of the right elbow of a 40-year-old man with quadriplegia, with heterotopic ossification limiting elbow range of motion.

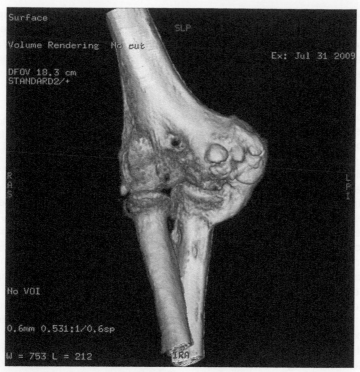

Fig. 13. Computed tomography demonstrating heterotopic ossification.

stability of the ulnohumeral joint is insufficient the soft tissues will ultimately yield. DIA continues to yield imperfect results; however, the coupling of hinged external fixation with interposition is an improvement over either technique in isolation.

CONTRACTURE RELEASE/EXCISION OF HETEROTOPIC OSSIFICATION

The release of elbow contracture or excision of heterotopic ossification often requires extensive release of capsuloligamentous structures that

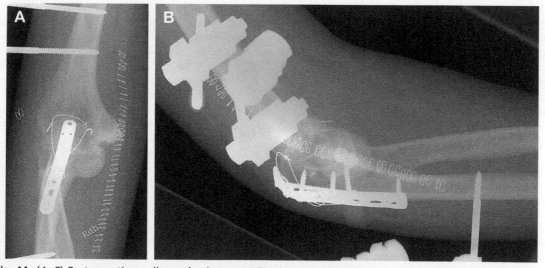

Fig. 14. (*A, B*) Postoperative radiographs demonstrating intraoperative fracture due to severe osteopenia. The olecranon fracture has been repaired with a locking plate and tension band. This was deemed insufficient in light of the severe osteopenia, and a hinged external fixator was applied.

can occasionally result in postoperative instability. In addition, loss of motion early in the postoperative period is frequent.[18] The rationale for hinged external fixator use in patients with severe elbow contracture or heterotopic ossification undergoing release is (1) to provide stability following extensive release and (2) to increase motion because of an increased ability to implement early motion and static progressive stretching.

Instability is a potential problem in these cases. The contracture is often posttraumatic. Occasionally, the collateral ligaments may be insufficient to maintain stability and this instability may be revealed after contracture release. In cases of heterotopic bone excision, the collateral ligaments are sometimes ossified. Excision of the collateral ligaments may also result in an unstable elbow.

However, it is unclear whether hinged external fixation improves range of motion after contracture release. Ring and colleagues[19] conducted a nonrandomized study of 42 patients undergoing operative release of severe posttraumatic elbow contracture and examined whether fixator placement affected final range of motion. Twenty-three patients were treated with a hinged external fixator after the procedure to apply static progressive stretch. The investigators found no statistically significant difference between groups treated with and without the external fixation. At present, the evidence favors using external fixation only with instability following contracture release or excision of heterotopic ossification.

Figs. 12–14 illustrate a case of heterotopic ossification in a 40-year-old quadriplegic man after a traumatic brain injury. Two years after injury, he had heterotopic bone encompassing the medial side of the elbow, including the medial collateral ligament (see **Figs. 12** and **13**). During excision, his olecranon fractured. The bone was osteoporotic and had tenuous fixation even with a locking construct augmented with tension banding. To protect the fracture repair and to prevent postresection instability, a Synthes Arm hinged external fixator was placed (see **Fig. 14**).

SUMMARY

Hinged external fixation of the elbow maintains concentric reduction of the joint while allowing early postoperative motion. Application requires particular attention to the axis of rotation of the ulnohumeral joint. The most common indications for a hinged external fixator are acute or chronic instability of the elbow after trauma, DIA, or use after contracture release or excision of heterotopic ossification.

Although situations requiring a hinged external fixator are uncommon, orthopedic surgeons should be familiar with how to apply a hinged fixator when faced with an unstable ulnohumeral joint despite addressing the bony and soft tissue constraints of the elbow.

ACKNOWLEDGMENTS

Thanks to Kristi Overgaard and April Schauer for their assistance in the preparation of this article.

REFERENCES

1. Mehlhoff TL, Noble PC, Bennett JB, et al. Simple dislocation of the elbow in the adult. Results after closed treatment. J Bone Joint Surg Am 1988; 70(2):244–9.
2. Morrey BF. Elbow biomechanics. In: Morrey BF, editor. The elbow and its disorders. Philadelphia: WB Saunders; 1985.
3. Morrey BF, Askew LJ, An KN, et al. A biomechanical study of normal functional elbow motion. J Bone Joint Surg Am 1981;63:872–7.
4. Madey SM, Bottlang M, Steyers CM, et al. Hinged external fixation of the elbow: Optimal alignment to minimize motion resistance. J Orthop Trauma 2000;14:41–7.
5. Behrens F. General theory and principles of external fixation. Clin Orthop 1989;241:15–23.
6. Behrens F, Johnson WD. Unilateral external fixation: methods to increase and reduce frame stiffness. Clin Orthop 1989;241:48–56.
7. Kamineni S, Hirahara H, Neale P, et al. Effectiveness of the lateral unilateral dynamic external fixator after elbow ligament injury. J Bone Joint Surg Am 2007; 89(8):1802–9.
8. Sekiya H, Neale PG, O'Driscoll SW, et al. An in vitro biomechanical study of a hinged external fixator applied to an unstable elbow. J Shoulder Elbow Surg 2005;14(4):429–32.
9. Stavlas P, Gliatis J, Polyzois V, et al. Unilateral hinged external fixator of the elbow in complex elbow injuries. Injury 2004;35(11):1158–66.
10. Ruch DS, Triepel CR. Hinged elbow fixation for recurrent instability following fracture dislocation. Injury 2001;32(Suppl 4):SD70–8.
11. McKee MD, Bowden SH, King GJ, et al. Management of recurrent, complex instability of the elbow with a hinged external fixator. J Bone Joint Surg Br 1998;80(6):1031–6.
12. Yu JR, Throckmorton TW, Bauer RM, et al. Management of acute complex instability of the elbow with hinged external fixation. J Shoulder Elbow Surg 2007;16(1):60–7.
13. Duckworth AD, Ring D, Kulijdian A, et al. Unstable elbow dislocations. J Shoulder Elbow Surg 2008; 17(2):281–6.

14. Jupiter JB, Ring D. Treatment of unreduced elbow dislocations with hinged external fixation. J Bone Joint Surg Am 2002;84(9):1630–5.

15. Morrey BF. Post-traumatic contracture of the elbow: operative treatment, including distraction arthroplasty. J Bone Joint Surg Am 1990;72:601–8.

16. Nolla J, Ring D, Lozano-Calderon S, et al. Interposition arthroplasty of the elbow with hinged external fixation for post-traumatic arthritis. J Shoulder Elbow Surg 2008;17(3):459–64.

17. Cheng SL, Morrey BF. Treatment of the mobile, painful arthritic elbow by distraction interposition arthroplasty. J Bone Joint Surg Am 2000;82(2):233–8.

18. Tan V, Daluiski A, Simic P, et al. Outcome of open release for post-traumatic elbow stiffness. J Trauma 2006;61(3):673–8.

19. Ring D, Hotchkiss RN, Guss D, et al. Hinged elbow external fixation for severe elbow contracture. J Bone Joint Surg Am 2005;87(6):1293–6.

The Role of Nerve Allografts and Conduits for Nerve Injuries

Michael Rivlin, MD[a], Emran Sheikh, MD[b,*], Roman Isaac, MD[c], Pedro K. Beredjiklian, MD[b,*]

KEYWORDS
- Conduit • Nerve repair • Nerve injury • Allograft
- Nerve gap • Nerve graft

Improvements in surgical techniques, instruments, and implant materials have opened new horizons in restoring and repairing injured nerves. Although numerous advances have been made to further understand nerve repair, regaining function of a nerve that has been injured is still highly variable and often unpredictable.[1] Nerve damage requiring surgical repair can occur after traumatic injuries, from purposeful surgical sacrifice following tumor resection, or from iatrogenic injury during surgery. About 3% of trauma patients in Level I trauma centers have a significant peripheral nerve injury, of which the radial nerve is the most commonly injured nerve (53%), followed by the ulnar (32%) and median nerves (15%).[2]

Although surgical repair of injured nerves with the use of microvascular techniques is well established, the treatment of injuries in which there is a gap at the repair site remains a challenge. Traditionally, autologous nerve or vein grafts have been used to bridge gaps between the nerve endings and have been the gold standard in nerve reconstruction surgery.[3] With the advancement of nerve restoration techniques, there are other options available for nerve reconstruction in this setting. The goal of this review article is to explore the role of nerve allografts and conduits in peripheral nerve reconstruction.

NERVE INJURY
Classification of Injury

Regardless of the mechanism of injury, nerve injuries are classified by anatomic extent of the damage. Seddon and colleagues[4] classified nerve injuries into neurapraxia (conduction defect without structural discontinuity), axonotmesis (loss of continuity of the axon), and neurotmesis (nerve disruption) (**Table 1**). Sunderland[5] further expanded this classification based on the microscopic features of Seddon and colleagues' observations. He described the importance of connective tissue changes, in particular the involvement of the endoneurium and its effect on recovery. Hence, he further classified the injuries into 5 types by histologic findings and explored how they directly relate to prognosis. Type 1 injury is the equivalent of neurapraxia in Seddon and colleagues' classification. Types 2 and 3 describe axonotmesis with intact endoneurium and axonotmesis with severed endoneurium respectively. In type 4 injury, both the endoneurium, as well as the perineurium are damaged. When all layers are disrupted, including the epineurium, the injury is classified as type 5, equivalent to neurotmesis. Although these classifications are difficult to correlate with each patient's presentation and therefore hard to apply in the clinical setting, they are

[a] Department of Orthopaedics, Thomas Jefferson University Hospital, 1015 Walnut Street, Curtis Building, Room 801, Philadelphia, PA 19107, USA
[b] Division of Hand Surgery, Rothman Institute, Thomas Jefferson University Hospital, 925 Chestnut Street, Philadelphia, PA 19107, USA
[c] Department of Orthopaedics, New York Medical College, St Vincent's Hospital, 170 West 12th Street, New York, NY 10011, USA
* Corresponding authors.

Hand Clin 26 (2010) 435–446
doi:10.1016/j.hcl.2010.04.010
0749-0712/10/$ – see front matter © 2010 Elsevier Inc. All rights reserved.

Table 1
Classification of nerve injury

Seddon's Classification	Sunderland's Classification	Anatomic Extent of the Injury	Spontaneous Recovery
Neurapraxia	1	None (conduction block)	Complete in hours to weeks
Axonotmesis	2	Axonal discontinuity	Complete in months
	3	Axonal discontinuity with endoneurial disruption	
	4	Axonal discontinuity with endoneurial and perineurial disruption	
Neurotmesis	5	Axonal discontinuity with endoneurial, perineurial and epineurial disruption	Negligible

good prognostic indicators for nerve recovery.[6] Sunderland[5] also described the expected recovery of various injuries. Complete or near complete recovery can be expected in type 1 and 2 injuries, with time frame ranging from hours to weeks in type 1 injuries and up to several months in type 2 injuries. With type 3 and 4 injuries, recovery usually does not lead to a degree of meaningful nerve function without surgical intervention. Likewise, useful spontaneous recovery is negligible in type 5 injuries.

Degeneration

After axonal transection, changes occur at the site of injury and to components proximal and distal to it. At the proximal zone of injury the nerve fiber undergoes degenerative changes. The extent of degeneration can range from affecting the nearest Node of Ranvier to global neuronal death depending on the nature and energy of the injury.[7]

After the injury, the neuron body swells and undergoes chromatolysis indicating a switch from active function to repair phase.[6] Schwann cell degradation, as well as a decrease in the diameter of the axon and myelin sheath, occurs at the site of injury and extends proximally. Perineural glial cells interrupt synapse connections of the neuron disconnecting it from the neural circuit.

Macrophages and Schwann cells play an important role in degeneration of the distal end of the nerve fiber, also known as Wallerian degeneration. The axonal microtubules and neurofilaments undergo proteolysis by a calcium-dependent process mediated by an axonal enzyme.[8] In response to local chemotaxis, macrophages and Schwann cells phagocytose myelin and axonal remnants.[9,10] After the process of degeneration is completed, Schwann cells realign themselves to form Bands of Büngner. These become the supportive leading structure for the regenerating axon distal to the site of injury. In types 3, 4, and 5 injuries, there is proliferation of the perineurial and endoneurial fibroblasts, which result in fibrous tissue. This scar may create a blockage and prevent regeneration of the axon distally, in effect interrupting the healing process.

Regeneration

Nerve regeneration varies upon the extent of the injury. In neurapraxia, there is only restoration of conduction ability. In axonotmesis and neurotmesis, where there is an anatomic disruption, regeneration involves anatomic and functional changes. The regenerative process usually begins after the Wallerian degeneration is complete; however, in less severe injuries, there is some overlap between the two processes.[6]

The earliest sign of regeneration is the reversal of chromatolysis. There is fluid accumulation and the formation of fibrin matrix between nerve endings.[11] This acellular process creates a supporting structure for the regenerating axon to bridge through the site of injury. Nerve growth factor (NGF) was the first neurotrophic factor to be described and isolated.[12] Normally, neurotrophic factors are synthesized by the nerve's end organ and transported back via the axon; however, after axonotomy, the neuronal cell lacks these factors.[13] Local macrophages up-regulate the production of NGF by Schwann cells by releasing IL-1.[14] Schwann cells, which are already in the vicinity following the degenerative reaction, are also responsible for manufacturing other trophic factors including insulin-like growth factor 1,[15] ciliary neurotrophic factor (CNTF),[16] and brain-derived neurotrophic factor (BDNF).[17] Other neurotrophic factors are postulated to play a role such as fibroblast growth factor, glial growth factor, and brain-derived growth factor, among others.[18]

In hours to weeks after injury, the axons sprout from the proximal end. At each regenerating axonal tip, the growth cone, lamelipodia (sheets of cell matrix), and filopodia (rich in actin) are guided toward basal lamina (fibronectin and laminin) via electrophilic interactions.[7,19] Fibronectin and laminin of Schwann cell basal lamina attract filopodia via electrophilic interactions. This process continues until the axons reach their end organ. The rate of axonal growth is assumed to be approximately 1 mm per day; however, the rate of growth is highly variable clinically.[5] In injuries where the endoneurial tube is disrupted, axon sprouts may grow into scar tissue, or other functionally inappropriate endoneurial tube, such as a neuroma. This interruption halts the development of the axon, and leads to permanent nerve dysfunction.

NERVE REPAIR
End-to-End Repair

The goal of surgical repair is to provide the framework for axonal growth. A number of options and techniques have been developed over the years, each with specific indications and limitations. Surgical options to connect severed nerve stumps anatomically include direct end-to-end and end-to-side neurorrhaphy, nerve grafting, and nerve transfers.

Primary repair is defined as direct end-to-end suture of separated nerve ends several days after injury. It is most favorable in sharp transections, with adequate vascularized nerve bed and clean wounds. The most important predictor of good outcome in end-to-end suture repair is small nerve gap with tensionless repair; multiple studies have shown a reduction in blood flow of approximately 50% when nerves are stretched to 10%.[20,21] Driscoll and colleagues[21] concluded that elongation to about 15% causes irreversible ischemic damage to nerves. Historically, primary nerve repair was performed 3 weeks after initial injury to provide time for Wallerian degeneration. In studies by Mackinnon,[22] better outcomes were found with early reconnection of transected nerve.

End-to-end repair includes epineurial and fascicular repair. Epineurial closure involves placing several nonabsorbable sutures in the epineurium of the free nerve ends. Care is taken to align the fascicles, which can be confirmed by vasa nervorum within the epineurium.[23] In distal nerve injuries, where the axons are grouped roughly by function, and the diameter of nerves are much smaller, epineurial repair is preferred.[24,25]

Fasicular repair involves dissection of the epineurium and suturing of the fascicles of same function together. This repair is useful in proximal nerve injury where the fascicles are easily identified and aligned, leading to decrease in misdirection of regenerating axons. However, extensive dissection and high number of suture requirements as compared with epineural repair can lead to increased scarring and diminished intraneural blood flow.[26,27]

End-to-Side Repair

End-to-Side (ETS) nerve repair offers an option for injuries of significant nerve gaps or irreversible damage to proximal nerve stumps. The basic neurobiological concept relies on nerve fiber regeneration along the distal stump of a transected nerve by inducing collateral axonal sprouting from a healthy neighbor donor nerve.[28] ETS techniques have traditionally included a lateral incision through the epineurium on the donor nerve with attachment of the distal stump of the injured one. In the early 1990s, Viterbo and colleagues[29] introduced a modified end-to-side neurorrhaphy without incision and injury to donor nerve and demonstrated promising results in a rat model. Some data have suggested that sensory axons may sprout without deliberately injuring the nerve sheaths of donor nerves, whereas motor axons regenerate only in response to a deliberate injury.[30] Experimental and clinical experience with ETS neurorrhaphy has rendered mixed results. Although continued clinical and laboratory experimentation with ETS nerve repair is warranted, it should not yet replace more established techniques of nerve repair.

Nerve Graft

In some cases the 2 nerve endings cannot be coaptated without tension, leading to gapping at the repair site. One option in this setting is the use of autologous nerve grafting. Nerve grafts, if performed in a tensionless manner, have been shown to generally have better results than an end-to-end approximation performed under tension.[31,32] There remains controversy about the best treatment options for small to moderate size nerve gaps. Extensive mobilization of nerve tissue and coaptation with mild tension carries the risk of decreased blood flow and proliferation of scar tissue.[31] Scar formation can block axonal regeneration and lead to neuroma formation.

For nerve defects exceeding 3 cm, nerve grafting is a viable option. Autologous nerve grafts fulfill the criteria for an ideal nerve conduit because they provide a permissive and stimulating scaffold including Schwann cell, basal laminae, neurotrophic factors, and adhesion molecules.[33] Common donor sites for autologous grafts are cutaneous sensory nerves, which provide acceptable morbidity in the form of noncritical sensory loss. Donor nerves include the sural nerve, lateral antebrachial cutaneous nerve, anterior division of the medial antebrachial cutaneous nerve, dorsal cutaneous branch of the ulnar nerve, and superficial sensory branch of the radial nerve.[34] To choose the best autologous nerve graft, one must take into consideration the caliber of the nerve to be repaired, length of the defect, and donor site.

In a trunk graft technique, a large section of a nerve is used to bridge the graft completely. This was similar to the cable grafts developed slightly later, in which smaller nerves were harvested and glued together to create a single large graft. Both of these methods resulted in little success.[35] The diameter and vascularity of the nerve graft are the most important factors influencing axonal outgrowth. Nonvascularized autografts survive by the diffusion from the surrounding tissues, and as a result of the direct capillary in-growth from the periphery and nerve ends, leading to nerve revascularization.[33,36] Application of thicker nerve grafts carries the risk of central necrosis and scar formation because of the poor diffusion and delayed revascularization.[37] Similarly, poorly vascularized tissue bed increases scar formation, delays nerve regeneration, and worsens functional outcome.[33] Many different types of grafting have been performed; however, outcomes are often unpredictable and highly variable.

ALLOGRAFTS

An alternative to autograft for repairs with gapping at the injury site include cadaveric allograft. With the advancement of tissue reprocessing and established tissue bank networks, the availability of high-quality autografts is on the rise. There are several theoretical and clinical advantages of these grafts compared with autografts. First, these grafts are readily available for implantation. Second, donor site morbidity (persistent pain, prolonged sensory loss, or neuroma formation) and operative time are significantly decreased.[38]

Cadaveric allografts can provide an adequate environment for axon regeneration. Fresh allografts have been used for nerve reconstruction but require an 18-month-long course of immunosuppression for the tissues to incorporate.[3,38] FK506(tacrolimus) and other immunosuppressive agents have been used for this purpose.[38] In the absence of immunosuppression, increased scarring and fibrosis from host rejection will likely impose a mechanical barrier for reinnervation.[38,39] Immunosuppressive agents that decrease the possibility of rejection carry the inherent risk of infection, decreased wound healing, and other systemic effects.

Processed allografts prevent a host reaction to the implant by removing the immunogenic constituents of the graft. Even though these grafts are decellularized and in the process lose important growth promoting elements such as Schwann cells and growth factors, they retain the internal scaffold, laminin, and other structural extracellular components that are important for regeneration. Hudson and colleagues[40] demonstrated that a processed (optimized acellular) nerve graft showed regeneration that was comparable to clinical isografts without the risk of immunogenic complications.

There are several ways of making cadaveric tissue biologically inert. By processing the donor specimen with chemicals, radiation, or with subjecting it to temperature extremes, the immunogenic properties of the implant can be decreased.[41] One such commercially available product is created by taking cadaveric nerves of various calibers and processed by a combination of detergent decellularization, chondroitinase chondroitin sulfate proteoglycan degradation, and gamma-irradiation sterilization.[42] The final product is a scaffold made of extracellular matrix.

In a rat model, Whitlock and colleagues[42] compared the regeneration of transected sciatic nerves using human decellularized allograft (Avance, AxogGen, Alachua, FL, USA), type 1 collagen conduit (NeuraGen, Integra, Plainsboro, NJ, USA), and isografts. The results show comparable outcomes of all groups long term in a short gap model (14 mm). However, in a long gap model of 28 mm, the results were divergent. Isografts performed best followed by the allograft group.

To augment the nerve regeneration process, cytokines have been added within the allograft to stimulate nerve growth. In one study, nerve growth factor (NGF) containing microspheres were fixed around processed grafts to aid axon regrowth.[43] Comparable morphologic results were achieved to autografts using this slow release growth-stimulating biologic construct.

Schwann cells were used by Wang and colleagues[44] to enhance regeneration. Autologous bone marrow stromal cells were introduced into the allogeneic nerve grafts before implantation in an animal model.[44] This modification favorably influenced nerve regeneration compared with allografts without bone marrow additive. Walsh and colleagues[45] introduced skin-derived precursor cells by injecting them in acellular nerve grafts in a rodent model. The precursor cells were predifferentiated toward a Schwann cell phenotype in vitro. After injecting these cells into acellular isografts, favorable results were observed compared with controls.

NERVE CONDUITS

In the search of alternatives to autografts and allo-grafts to bridge nerve gaps, commercially manu-factured natural and synthetic conduits have recently gained attention. In contrast with auto or allograft nerve materials, the obvious advantages of nerve repairs with conduits include avoidance of donor site morbidity and problems associated with immunosuppression. In addition, repair with a conduit creates an isolated environment by en-veloping the repair site and the distal and proximal ends of the nerve. This milieu helps to contain the needed cytokines necessary for nerve regenera-tion, and sets up the needed gradient of molecular signaling molecules. In addition, the barrier created by this artificial environment protects the repair site from fibroblast and inflammatory cell penetration. Furthermore, these constructs prevent any mechanical obstacle from intruding between the regenerating nerve ends and guides the axon sprouts to their counterparts. In 1964, Kline and Hayes[46] wrapped the primarily sutured nerve ends in a collagen sheet in a primate model and showed increased organization of micro-scopic structures. It was not until later that enclos-ing nerves with a gap in between was attempted.

Pathophysiology of Nerve Conduits

Research has been performed in an effort to understand the physiologic events that occur within the entubulated regenerating nerve construct. After the implantation of the conduit, immediate changes take place. Fluid is excreted from the nerve ends, setting up a gradient of neu-rotrophic factors to guide the cells toward the opposite side.[47] Next, a fibrin matrix appears in coaxial orientation within the first week of regener-ation.[48] This creates scaffolding for the cells that aids the axonal growth. During the second week, with the help of Schwann cells and other supportive cells, myelinated, as well as unmyelin-ated, nerve fibers begin to cross the gap in direct line toward the opposite end.[49] As more and more axon sprouts reach the opposing terminal, a superstructure of fibers emerges. By the end of the sixth week, nerve fibers have matured and the disappearance of macrophages indicates the completion of the nerve regeneration (as demon-strated in a 5-mm gap).[49]

Conduit Materials and Designs

Several biomaterials have been used to create the optimal tubular structure for a nerve conduit. Synthetic and natural, permanent, and absorbable tubes have been implanted, using tubes made

from glass, metal, bone, muscle, connective tissues, veins, and bioengineered materials.[50]

One of the original conduits used for treatment of traumatic nerve injuries was a vein graft. These offer the advantage of minimal donor site morbidity, abundant availability, and no associ-ated cost of grafts. In addition, because these grafts are autografts, the risk of immunogenic reaction is eliminated, preventing rejection. Even though the disadvantages of these autografts are not well described, harvest complications and free-flow impeding valves may hinder their perfor-mance. Lee and Shieh[51] have shown that vein grafts perform well at reconstructing digital sensory nerves. At 10-year follow-up they demon-strated 3 cases with excellent outcomes (3–3+, Modified Highet and Sander criteria).[52] When compared with direct repair, vein grafts have less predictable and often inferior outcome; however, this technique has shown some clinical merit in nonessential sensory nerve reconstructions in the upper extremity.[53] Although the maximum gap distance that is amenable to vein graft repair has not been clinically established, animal studies demonstrated that gap lengths of greater than 3 cm become less predictable, with longer defects, outcomes become increasingly poor.[54]

Silicone was one of the first nonabsorbable synthetic nerve conduits that was used for bridging a nerve gap. It offers reliable material properties with versatile physical characteristics used in many other surgical devices and implants. In one of the first demonstrations of how a conduit may promote nerve growth, Lundborg and colleagues[55] described the reinervation patterns between nerve stumps in a microenvironment of silicone chambers in a rodent model. Further investigations revealed up to 80% recovery of rat sciatic nerve defects, a result that was comparable with conventional nerve grafts.[56] In a case-controlled prospective study, these investigators observed essentially no difference in the regener-ation of 3- to 4-mm nerve gaps compared with primary microsurgical repair of human median and ulnar nerves. The only difference between groups was in the sensory modality of touch at 3-month follow-up in favor of the experimental group.[57] These observations showed promise for the future of synthetic, nonabsorbable nerve graft substitutes. The main disadvantage of silicone conduits, as well as other nonbioabsorbable implants, is that they have to be explanted after integration (usually after 4 months, but occasion-ally up to 1 year after they are implanted).[58]

In recent years, the practicality of using nonab-sorbable tubules has come into question. Dhalin and Lundborg[59] evaluated silicone grafts at the time of explantation at 1 year follow-up. The investigators found that the grafts were surrounded by a thin line of mesothelial layer. This reaction was thought to contribute to the compressive effects of the conduits, which is thought to adversely affect nerve function. Furthermore, they believed that this encapsulation with mesothelial lining may offer more protection and allow gliding of the construct, thereby reducing trauma to the regenerating nerves. This study revealed no compression of nerve ends and demonstrated good outcomes of bridging small nerve gaps of the medial and ulnar nerves. Because these implants are permanent and do not get reabsorbed by the host, local effects often adversely affect their outcomes.

Polyglycolic acid (PGA) has been purported as a potential absorbable biomaterial for use in nerve conduits. This biodegradable thermo-polymer is the main component of commonly used suture material, Dexon (Syneture) or Vicryl (Ethicon). Therefore, it has a long track record of safety in clinical use.

The advantage of PGA is that it breaks down reliably in vitro via simple hydrolytic reactions. After implantation, it takes approximately 90 days to degrade and get absorbed.[19] In 1986, Merrell and colleagues[60] used PGA conduit in an animal model and demonstrated clinically equivalent results to direct suture technique. Mackinon and Dellon[61] devoted much attention to evaluate the clinical effectiveness of PGA conduits first in animal then in human subjects.[62] In monkeys, these investigators compared the regeneration across a short nerve gap (3 cm) using PGA conduit and interfascicular interpositional sural nerve graft. Even though the nerve diameters and conduction velocities were lower than those in the control group, electrophysiological and microscopic evaluation demonstrated nerve regeneration in all experimental groups.[62] In a similar study, the investigators implanted PGA conduits in 15 patients with nerve gaps of 0.5 to 3.0 cm and followed their function for an average of 2 years. [61] They found that 33% of the subjects achieved excellent functional sensation, and 53% achieved good functional sensation in their evaluation using 2-point discrimination as the outcome variable. Weber and colleagues[1] performed a randomized prospective study comparing standard repair using end-to-end neurorrhaphy or autograft reconstruction, compared with nerve conduit repair. The investigators found no significant difference between the 2 groups: patients with standard repair achieved good to excellent outcomes in 86% of cases, compared with 74% in the experimental group. The investigators noted that patients with gaps smaller than 4 mm benefited from conduit repair compared with those treated with the standard technique.

As the search for ideal nerve conduit continues, other natural and synthetic materials have been used. Because of its adaptive features and biologically friendly attributes, collagen has received some attention. Archibald and colleagues[63,64] demonstrated the use of highly purified type I collagen as a nerve guide in rodents and primates with promising results. The investigators compared the regeneration of 5-mm nerve gaps in primate median nerves using direct suture repair, autografts, and conduits. Their data showed that regeneration was similar between the autograft and conduit repair as demonstrated by electrophysiological assessment. The investigators concluded that conduit repair was physiologically equivalent to autograft and primary suture techniques. Further studies have shown that these constructs are viable alternatives in larger gaps; however, limitations have been found in the gap length that can be successfully repaired by conduits. This finding is attributable to the strict temporal relationship between the speed of axon growth from the stump and the time to traverse the gap.[65] In humans, a case series demonstrated good to excellent outcome in most patients with no reported adverse events attributable to the conduits themselves.[66] Collagen conduits are also available in mesh form that is designed to aid regeneration and protect nerves by wrapping the affected areas. Nurawrap (Integra) is used for peripheral nerve injuries without significant nervous tissue loss. It may offer additional support over a primary tensionless neurorrhaphy (**Fig. 1**).

In comparison with other conduit materials, collagen tubes appear to offer some advantage clinically, although there is not enough equivocal evidence found in the literature. Waitayawinyu and colleagues[67] compared PGA and collagen repair with autografts in a rat model. The investigators found that collagen conduits and autografts produced comparable results. In contrast, the PGA group showed inferior parameters in muscle contraction force, axonal counts, and wet muscle weight, and showed axons in a less organized orientation. Another animal study that compared the use of autografts to poly-DL-lactide-e-caprolactone, collagen, and PGA conduits demonstrated similar results.[68] PGA conduits were found to be collapsed at week 12 rendering them nonfunctional and preventing adequate regeneration. Even though collagen conduits showed significantly better outcomes compared with PGA, they were still inferior compared with autografts and poly-DL-lactide-e-caprolactone guides.

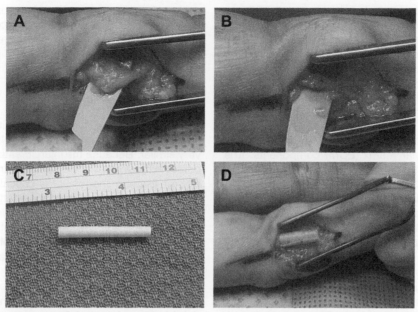

Fig. 1. Patient with painful neuroma formation between 2 nerve ends 6 weeks after laceration of the ring finger ulnar digital nerve. (*A*) The neruoma dissected. (*B*) The neuroma excised and primary tensionless neurorrhaphy performed. (*C*) Neurawrap (Integra) collagen conduit. (*D*) The digital nerve is enclosed in the appropriately sized Neurawrap (Integra).

When comparing processed allografts to collagen conduit in an animal study, Whitlock and colleagues[42] evaluated both functional and histomorphometric outcomes. Their findings show that in a short nerve gap model, outcomes are equivalent at long term between allografts and autografts (at short term, allografts appear to be incorporated at a faster rate). On the other hand, allografts present superior outcomes in a long nerve gap model (28 mm). This difference was significant in all points of evaluation, apparent both by histomorphometry analysis and functional analysis.

Another synthetic conduit that has received attention in animal studies is made of fibrin. Fibrin glue conduits have been proposed as a biodegradable nonimmunogenic alternative to conventional conduits. In animal studies the outcomes were promising compared with controls, but further studies are required before their use clinically.[69]

There are no large nerve conduit prospective randomized studies published on humans at the time of writing this article. However, from our understanding of animal studies as well as clinical outcome studies, collagen conduits appear to hold strong promise as an alternative to autograft repair.

Luminal Fillers

To promote faster and more functional nerve regeneration, recent research is looking into adding growth-promoting factors, structural matrix components, and glial cells into nerve conduits. A number of animal studies show promising results in using them as luminal fillers. After nerve injury, neurotrophic factors, extracellular matrix, and cellular signals are released from nerve ends, which are vital for differentiation and regeneration of nervous tissue. Latest research is looking into promoting the optimal conduit environment by introducing these factors.

Neurotrophic factors such as NGF, fibroblast nerve factor (FGF), and glial growth factor (GGF) are vital for nerve repair. NGF plays an important role in natural process of nerve regeneration and growth. In treatment of a 5-mm sciatic nerve injury in rats, motor nerve conduction velocities increased after introduction of NGF solution into silicone nerve conduit.[70] Rich and colleagues[71] showed similar results with introduction of NGF into rat sciatic nerve models. Their results showed doubling of the number of axons in conduit, and the myelin sheath increased in thickness when compared with normal saline. FGFs are a family of cytokines that stimulate mitogenesis in a wide variety of cell types following injury to peripheral nerves.[72] An acidic FGF incorporated into collagen-filled nerve conduits increased formation of myelinated axons across a 5-mm sciatic nerve defect of a rat as compared with control groups.[73] GGF stimulates proliferation of Schwann cells.

Mohanna and colleagues,[74] introduced GGF into conduits attached to rabbit peroneal nerve gaps, which showed an increase in the number of Schwann cells and the rate of axonal regeneration. Among other neurotrophic factors are neurotropin-3 (NT-3) and brain-derived neurotrophic factor (BDNF), which have both been shown to increase rat sciatic nerve regeneration in a synthetic hydrogel tube.[75]

A number of studies also looked into the role of the extracellular matrix (ECM) components. It is well known that after a nerve is transected it secretes ECM molecules, mainly fibronectin, collagen, and laminin, which are used as scaffold for cells to aggregate and regenerate neuronal tissue.[48] Whitworth and colleagues[76] used fibronectin mats as nerve conduits to bridge a 10-mm sciatic nerve defect in rats. The fibronectin group showed a faster rate of axonal growth compared with muscle grafts within first the 10 days. Furthermore, the same group showed a similar amount of regenerating axons and Schwann cells as compared with nerve grafts after 15 days of repair. Madison and colleagues[77] introduced laminin into a nerve conduit, bridging marine sciatic nerve, and showed promising results at 2 weeks. Their future experiments showed laminin significantly increases initial axonal regeneration, but at the same time inhibits the process at 6 weeks.[78] The use of collagen in a PGA conduit of a 5-mm rate peroneal defect showed axonal regeneration equal to sutured autografts at 12 months.[79]

The cellular components, such as Schwann cells, macrophages, and fibroblasts, aggregate on the extracellular matrix after nerve injury and are critical for nerve repair. Multiple studies show that the presence of Schwann cells results in improved nerve regeneration and functional outcome.[80,81] Cheng and Chen[82] introduced them into conduits to bridge a 20-mm gap of rat sciatic nerve. The number of axons and area of nerve fibers was comparable to the autograft group at 3 months. Schwann cells are difficult to obtain for the use of luminal fillers. An alternative is bone stromal cells, which are multipotent stem cells that have the ability to differentiate into neural cells. Zhang and colleagues[83] introduced both Schwann cells and bone stromal cells into biodegradable conduits using rat sciatic nerve conduits. Both groups showed a significantly higher number of axons, nerve conduction velocity, and sciatic functional index at 6 weeks as compared with the empty conduit group.

A number of animal studies show promising results in using a variety of luminal fillers in nerve conduits. Most inspiring are NGF and FGF results. The wide range of luminal fillers and versatile designs for incorporating them into nerve conduits are major advantages over autograft. New research is focusing on clinical applications, a combination of different fillers, and discovery of new, manufactured fillers.

OPERATIVE TECHNIQUE

Regardless of the type of conduit used, the surgical principle and steps of implantation are very similar. Because the injury creating the nerve defect is most often in the setting of trauma, careful soft tissue management is critical to promote the healing of the wound. Concomitantly, the healing potential of the nerve injury is equally maximized. In addition, because an implant is used, the appropriate prophylactic antibiotic coverage following thorough wound irrigation and debridement will help prevent infection.

After proper setup and surgical approach under tourniquet control, the affected region is explored, debrided, and irrigated. The nerve is isolated and freed to allow for manipulation with care to minimize devitalization. Because the nerve ends have to be viable, fresh, and penetrable by cells and the growing axons, they have to be prepared before the application of the conduit.[1] The nerve ends are trimmed back to where the tissue is healthy with no hematoma or interfascicular scarring apparent. It is important that good hemostasis is achieved at the nerve ends to prevent hematoma formation within the conduit. This can be checked by the temporary deflation of the tourniquet.

The tension-free gap distance is measured with the limb in neutral position. To determine the appropriate conduit, the diameter is measured. Collagen tubes, such as NeuraGen (Integra) nerve guides come in 2- and 3-cm lengths and diameters of 1.5 to 7.0 mm. PGA conduits, for example the Neurotube (Synovis, Birmingham, AL, USA), are supplied in the range of 2.3- to 8.0-mm diameters and 2- to 4-cm lengths.

Using 8-0 to 10-0 nylon suture, 2 or more epineural stitches are applied (**Fig. 2**). By securing the sutures in a horizontal mattress configuration, the nerve ends are pulled into the tube. It is recommended that 5 mm of the nerve is encapsulated by the conduit on each end for stability and good seal.[1] The minimum distance between ends is 5 mm.

The intraluminal space is filled with the solution recommended by the manufacturer. Collagen tubes are filled with saline. The recommendation for the PGA tubes on the other hand is heparinized saline (10 units per milliliter) to prevent clot formation within the construct.

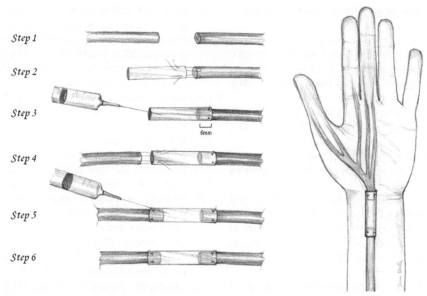

Fig. 2. Major steps of conduit implantation (*left*): Step 1 – prepared nerve ends, Step 2 – suturing of the conduit to the nerve stump, Step 3 – filling the conduit, Step 4 – suturing the opposite end of the nerve in place, Step 5 – topping off the intraluminal fluid, Step 6 – enclosed nerve. Schematic representation of nerve conduit in vitro (*right*). (*Courtesy of* Anna Marfin.)

The opposing end of the nerve is sutured and pulled into the tube in a similar way as the first end. Additional sutures may be added to provide more stability. There is a final injection of solution into the tube to ensure that the conduit is filled. By preventing air bubbles, a more uniform gradient can be created by neurotrophic factors for the proper milieu required for axonal regeneration. Fibrin glue may be used as an additional material to isolate the internal environment from the external one. However, using sealants should not substitute for well-positioned and secure sutures.

The wound is irrigated and slack soft tissue coverage is attempted to avoid placing the repaired nerve directly subcutaneously. The nerve construct should sit loose, preferably in a low-stress position (away from joints, tendons, and ligaments). The wound is then closed and the extremity splinted in a protected position.

Postoperatively, a splint is used for protection of the repair for approximately 4 to 6 weeks. Thereafter, a course of physical or occupational therapy is usually needed to regain motion, strength, and function. The expectance of clinically observable nerve recovery is related to the distance of nerve injury from the target organ. Poor prognostic factors include large gap size, advanced patient age, substantial distance from the site of injury to the end organ, and injury to mixed (sensory and motor) nerves, among others.

SUMMARY

Treatment of nerve injuries, particularly those involving segmental nerve tissue loss leading to a gap between nerve endings, remains a vexing clinical problem. Commercially available nerve conduits can be helpful in the treatment of these patients. These conduits not only allow the regenerating axons to find the proper target, but also concentrate the neurotrophic factors and prevent axon escape through the suture gaps. Future advances in this area include the development of new biomaterials, identification of cytokines or growth factors that may enhance nerve regeneration, and the development of tissue-engineered nerve grafts.

ACKNOWLEDGMENTS

The authors thank Anna Marfin for her help with the figures included in this article.

REFERENCES

1. Weber RA, Breidenbach WC, Brown RE, et al. A randomized prospective study of polyglycolic acid conduits for digital nerve reconstruction in humans. Plast Reconstr Surg 2000;106(5):1036–45 [discussion: 1046–8].
2. Noble J, Munro CA, Prasad VS, et al. Analysis of upper and lower extremity peripheral nerve injuries

in a population of patients with multiple injuries. J Trauma 1998;45(1):116–22.

3. Mackinnon SE. Surgical management of the peripheral nerve gap. Clin Plast Surg 1989;16(3):587–603.

4. Seddon HJ, Medawar PB, Smith H. Rate of regeneration of peripheral nerves in man. J Physiol 1943; 102(2):191–215.

5. Sunderland S. Nerves and nerve injuries. 2nd edition. London: Churchill Livingstone; 1978. 120–127, 134–140.

6. Burnett MG, Zager EL. Pathophysiology of peripheral nerve injury: a brief review. Neurosurg Focus 2004;16(5):E1.

7. Lee SK, Wolfe SW. Peripheral nerve injury and repair. J Am Acad Orthop Surg 2000;8(4):243–52.

8. Schlaepfer WW, Hasler MB. Characterization of the calcium-induced disruption of neurofilaments in rat peripheral nerve. Brain Res 1979;168(2): 299–309.

9. Liu HM. Schwann cell properties. II. The identity of phagocytes in the degenerating nerve. Am J Pathol 1974;75(2):395–416.

10. Reichert F, Saada A, Rotshenker S. Peripheral nerve injury induces Schwann cells to express two macrophage phenotypes: phagocytosis and the galactose-specific lectin MAC-2. J Neurosci 1994;14(5 Pt 2):3231–45.

11. Williams LR, Longo FM, Powell HC, et al. Spatial-temporal progress of peripheral nerve regeneration within a silicone chamber: parameters for a bioassay. J Comp Neurol 1983;218(4):460–70.

12. Cohen S, Levi-Montalcini R, Hamburger V. A nerve growth-stimulating factor isolated from Sarcom as 37 and 180. Proc Natl Acad Sci U S A 1954; 40(10):1014–8.

13. Terenghi G. Peripheral nerve regeneration and neurotrophic factors. J Anat 1999;194(Pt 1):1–14.

14. Lindholm D, Heumann R, Meyer M, et al. Interleukin-1 regulates synthesis of nerve growth factor in nonneuronal cells of rat sciatic nerve. Nature 1987; 330(6149):658–9.

15. Hansson HA, Dahlin LB, Danielsen N, et al. Evidence indicating trophic importance of IGF-I in regenerating peripheral nerves. Acta Physiol Scand 1986;126(4):609–14.

16. Rende M, Muir D, Ruoslahti E, et al. Immunolocalization of ciliary neuronotrophic factor in adult rat sciatic nerve. Glia 1992;5(1):25–32.

17. Meyer M, Matsuoka I, Wetmore C, et al. Enhanced synthesis of brain-derived neurotrophic factor in the lesioned peripheral nerve: different mechanisms are responsible for the regulation of BDNF and NGF mRNA. J Cell Biol 1992;119(1):45–54.

18. Lundborg GA. 25-year perspective of peripheral nerve surgery: evolving neuroscientific concepts and clinical significance. J Hand Surg Am 2000; 25(3):391–414.

19. Weber RA, Dellon AL. Nerve lacerations: repair of acute injuries. In: Berger RA, Weiss AC, editors. Hand surgery. Philadelphia (PA): Lippincott Williams & Wilkins; 2004. p. 819–24, 833–834, Chapter 45.

20. Clark WL, Trumble TE, Swiontkowski MF, et al. Nerve tension and blood flow in a rat model of immediate and delayed repairs. J Hand Surg Am 1992;17(4):677–87.

21. Driscoll PJ, Glasby MA, Lawson GM. An in vivo study of peripheral nerves in continuity: biomechanical and physiological responses to elongation. J Orthop Res 2002;20(2):370–5.

22. Mackinnon SE. New directions in peripheral nerve surgery. Ann Plast Surg 1989;22(3):257–73.

23. Wilgis EF. Techniques of epineural and group fascicular repair. In: Gelberman RH, editor, In: Operative nerve repair and reconstruction, vol 1. Philadelphia: JB Lippincott; 1991. p. 287–93.

24. Diao E, Vannuyen T. Techniques for primary nerve repair. Hand Clin 2000;16(1):53–66, viii.

25. Jabaley ME, Wallace WH, Heckler FR. Internal topography of major nerves of the forearm and hand: a current view. J Hand Surg Am 1980;5(1):1–18.

26. Brushart TM, Tarlov EC, Mesulam MM. Specificity of muscle reinnervation after epineurial and individual fascicular suture of the rat sciatic nerve. J Hand Surg Am 1983;8(3):248–53.

27. Ogata K, Naito M. Blood flow of peripheral nerve effects of dissection, stretching and compression. J Hand Surg Br 1986;11(1):10–4.

28. Geuna S, Papalia I, Tos P. End-to-side (terminolateral) nerve regeneration: a challenge for neuroscientists coming from an intriguing nerve repair concept. Brain Res Rev 2006;52(2):381–8.

29. Viterbo F, Trindade JC, Hoshino K, et al. Lateroterminal neurorrhaphy without removal of the epineural sheath: experimental study in rats. Rev Paul Med 1992;110:267–75.

30. Pannucci C, Myckatyn TM, Mackinnon SE, et al. End-to-side nerve repair: review of the literature. Restor Neurol Neurosci 2007;25(1):45–63.

31. Terzis J, Faibisoff B, Williams B. The nerve gap: suture under tension vs. graft. Plast Reconstr Surg 1975;56(2):166–70.

32. Rodkey WG, Cabaud HE, McCarroll HR Jr. Neurorrhaphy after loss of a nerve segment: comparison of epineurial suture under tension versus multiple nerve grafts. J Hand Surg Am 1980; 5(4):366–71.

33. Almgren KG. Revascularization of free pheripheral nerve grafts. An experimental study in the rabbit. Acta Orthop Scand Suppl 1975;154:1–104.

34. Matsuyama T, Mackay M, Midha R. Peripheral nerve repair and grafting techniques: a review. Neurol Med Chir (Tokyo) 2000;40(4):187–99.

35. Wilgis EF. Nerve repair and grafting. In: Green DP, editor. 2nd edition, In: Operative hand surgery, vol. 2. New York: Churchill Livingstone; 1988. p. 1373–404.

36. Millesi H. Techniques for nerve grafting. Hand Clin 2000;16(1):73–91, viii.
37. Nunley JA. Donor nerves for grafting. In: Gelberman RH, editor, In: Operative nerve repair and reconstruction, vol. 1. Philadelphia: JB Lippincott; 1991. p. 545–52.
38. Mackinnon SE, Doolabh VB, Novak CB, et al. Clinical outcome following nerve allograft transplantation. Plast Reconstr Surg 2001;107(6):1419–29.
39. Rustemeyer J, van de Wal R, Keipert C, et al. Administration of low-dose FK 506 accelerates histomorphometric regeneration and functional outcomes after allograft nerve repair in a rat model. J Craniomaxillofac Surg 2009. [Epub ahead of print]. DOI:10.1016/j.jcms.2009.03.008.
40. Hudson TW, Zawko S, Deister C, et al. Optimized acellular nerve graft is immunologically tolerated and supports regeneration. Tissue Eng 2004; 10(11–12):1641–51.
41. Karabekmez FE, Duymaz A, Moran SL. Early clinical outcomes with the use of decellularized nerve allograft for repair of sensory defects within the hand. Hand (N Y) 2009;4(3):245–9.
42. Whitlock EL, Tuffaha SH, Luciano JP, et al. Processed allografts and type I collagen conduits for repair of peripheral nerve gaps. Muscle Nerve 2009;39(6):787–99.
43. Yu H, Peng J, Guo Q, et al. Improvement of peripheral nerve regeneration in acellular nerve grafts with local release of nerve growth factor. Microsurgery 2009;29(4):330–6.
44. Wang D, Liu XL, Zhu JK, et al. Bridging small-gap peripheral nerve defects using acellular nerve allograft implanted with autologous bone marrow stromal cells in primates. Brain Res 2008;1188:44–53.
45. Walsh S, Biernaskie J, Kemp SW, et al. Supplementation of acellular nerve grafts with skin derived precursor cells promotes peripheral nerve regeneration. Neuroscience 2009;164(3):1097–107.
46. Kline DG, Hayes GJ. The use of a resorbable wrapper for peripheral-nerve repair: experimental studies in chimpanzees. J Neurosurg 1964;21: 737–50.
47. Zheng M, Kuffler DP. Guidance of regenerating motor axons in vivo by gradients of diffusible peripheral nerve-derived factors. J Neurobiol 2000;42(2): 212–9.
48. Williams LR, Varon S. Modification of fibrin matrix formation in situ enhances nerve regeneration in silicone chambers. J Comp Neurol 1985;231(2): 209–20.
49. Li J, Yan JG, Ai X, et al. Ultrastructural analysis of peripheral-nerve regeneration within a nerve conduit. J Reconstr Microsurg 2004;20(7):565–9.
50. Hudson TW, Evans GR, Schmidt CE. Engineering strategies for peripheral nerve repair. Clin Plast Surg 1999;26(4):617–28, ix.
51. Lee YH, Shieh SJ. Secondary nerve reconstruction using vein conduit grafts for neglected digital nerve injuries. Microsurgery 2008;28(6):436–40.
52. Lee YH, Shieh SJ. Secondary nerve reconstruction using vein conduit grafts for neglected digital nerve injuries. Microsurgery 2008;28(6):436–40.
53. Chiu DT, Strauch B. A prospective clinical evaluation of autogenous vein grafts used as a nerve conduit for distal sensory nerve defects of 3 cm or less. Plast Reconstr Surg 1990;86(5):928–34.
54. Strauch B, Ferder M, Lovelle-Allen S, et al. Determining the maximal length of a vein conduit used as an interposition graft for nerve regeneration. J Reconstr Microsurg 1996;12(8):521–7.
55. Lundborg G, Longo FM, Varon S. Nerve regeneration model and trophic factors in vivo. Brain Res 1982;232(1):157–61.
56. Urabe T, Zhao Q, Danielsen N, et al. Regeneration across a partial defect in rat sciatic nerve encased in a silicone chamber. Scand J Plast Reconstr Surg Hand Surg 1996;30(1):7–15.
57. Lundborg G, Rosen B, Dahlin L, et al. Tubular versus conventional repair of median and ulnar nerves in the human forearm: early results from a prospective, randomized, clinical study. J Hand Surg Am 1997; 22(1):99–106.
58. Dellon AL. Use of a silicone tube for the reconstruction of a nerve injury. J Hand Surg Br 1994;19(3): 271–2.
59. Dahlin LB, Lundborg G. Use of tubes in peripheral nerve repair. Neurosurg Clin N Am 2001;12(2): 341–52.
60. Merrell JC, Russell RC, Zook EG. Polyglycolic acid tubing as a conduit for nerve regeneration. Ann Plast Surg 1986;17(1):49–58.
61. Mackinnon SE, Dellon AL. Clinical nerve reconstruction with a bioabsorbable polyglycolic acid tube. Plast Reconstr Surg 1990;85(3):419–24.
62. Dellon AL, Mackinnon SE. An alternative to the classical nerve graft for the management of the short nerve gap. Plast Reconstr Surg 1988;82(5): 849–56.
63. Archibald SJ, Krarup C, Shefner J, et al. A collagen-based nerve guide conduit for peripheral nerve repair: an electrophysiological study of nerve regeneration in rodents and nonhuman primates. J Comp Neurol 1991;306(4):685–96.
64. Archibald SJ, Shefner J, Krarup C, et al. Monkey median nerve repaired by nerve graft or collagen nerve guide tube. J Neurosci 1995;15(5 Pt 2): 4109–23.
65. Krarup C, Archibald SJ, Madison RD. Factors that influence peripheral nerve regeneration: an electrophysiological study of the monkey median nerve. Ann Neurol 2002;51(1):69–81.
66. Bushnell BD, McWilliams AD, Whitener GB, et al. Early clinical experience with collagen nerve tubes

in digital nerve repair. J Hand Surg Am 2008;33(7): 1081–7.

67. Waitayawinyu T, Parisi DM, Miller B, et al. A comparison of polyglycolic acid versus type 1 collagen bioabsorbable nerve conduits in a rat model: an alternative to autografting. J Hand Surg Am 2007; 32(10):1521–9.

68. Shin RH, Friedrich PF, Crum BA, et al. Treatment of a segmental nerve defect in the rat with use of bioabsorbable synthetic nerve conduits: a comparison of commercially available conduits. J Bone Joint Surg Am 2009;91(9):2194–204.

69. Pettersson J, Kalbermatten D, McGrath A, et al. Biodegradable fibrin conduit promotes long-term regeneration after peripheral nerve injury in adult rats. J Plast Reconstr Aesthet Surg 2009. [Epub ahead of print]. DOI:10.1016/j.bjps.2009.11.024.

70. He C, Chen Z, Chen Z. Enhancement of motor nerve regeneration by nerve growth factor. Microsurgery 1992;13(3):151–4.

71. Rich KM, Alexander TD, Pryor JC, et al. Nerve growth factor enhances regeneration through silicone chambers. Exp Neurol 1989;105(2):162–70.

72. Richardson PM. Neurotrophic factors in regeneration. Curr Opin Neurobiol 1991;1(3):401–6.

73. Cordeiro PG, Seckel BR, Lipton SA, et al. Acidic fibroblast growth factor enhances peripheral nerve regeneration in vivo. Plast Reconstr Surg 1989; 83(6):1013–9 [discussion: 1020–1].

74. Mohanna PN, Terenghi G, Wiberg M. Composite PHB-GGF conduit for long nerve gap repair: a long-term evaluation. Scand J Plast Reconstr Surg Hand Surg 2005;39(3):129–37.

75. Midha R, Munro CA, Dalton PD, et al. Growth factor enhancement of peripheral nerve regeneration through a novel synthetic hydrogel tube. J Neurosurg 2003;99(3):555–65.

76. Whitworth IH, Brown RA, Dore C, et al. Orientated mats of fibronectin as a conduit material for use in peripheral nerve repair. J Hand Surg Br 1995; 20(4):429–36.

77. Madison R, da Silva CF, Dikkes P, et al. Increased rate of peripheral nerve regeneration using bioresorbable nerve guides and a laminin-containing gel. Exp Neurol 1985;88(3):767–72.

78. Madison RD, da Silva C, Dikkes P, et al. Peripheral nerve regeneration with entubulation repair: comparison of biodegradable nerve guides versus polyethylene tubes and the effects of a laminin-containing gel. Exp Neurol 1987;95(2):378–90.

79. Rosen JM, Padilla JA, Nguyen KD, et al. Artificial nerve graft using collagen as an extracellular matrix for nerve repair compared with sutured autograft in a rat model. Ann Plast Surg 1990;25(5):375–87.

80. Koshimune M, Takamatsu K, Nakatsuka H, et al. Creating bioabsorbable Schwann cell coated conduits through tissue engineering. Biomed Mater Eng 2003;13(3):223–9.

81. Rodriguez FJ, Verdu E, Ceballos D, et al. Nerve guides seeded with autologous schwann cells improve nerve regeneration. Exp Neurol 2000; 161(2):571–84.

82. Cheng B, Chen Z. Fabricating autologous tissue to engineer artificial nerve. Microsurgery 2002;22(4): 133–7.

83. Zhang P, He X, Zhao F, et al. Bridging small-gap peripheral nerve defects using biodegradable chitin conduits with cultured schwann and bone marrow stromal cells in rats. J Reconstr Microsurg 2005; 21(8):565–71.

Three-Dimensional Computed Tomographic Imaging and Modeling in the Upper Extremity

Thierry G. Guitton, MSc, David Ring, MD, PhD*

KEYWORDS

- Computed tomography • Imaging • Modeling
- Upper extremity

Three-dimensional (3D) imaging has several potential advantages over radiographs and 2-dimensional (2D) computed tomography (CT).[1,2] Three-dimensional imaging is more intuitive, and structures look similar to what the surgeon sees in the operating room. In addition, the technique has been associated with improved identification of single fragments, articular surfaces, and fracture edges,[3] which allows better preoperative planning in terms of implants and equipment while also facilitating the surgeon's mental and psychomotor preparation. Three-dimensional imaging is also more intuitive for patients and could lead to better understanding and improved decision making and compliance.

There are several potential disadvantages of 3D imaging, which include increased cost and resource use to produce the images. In addition, the production of these images takes more time than that of a standard x-ray or CT images. This could be an issue in emergency cases.

Three-dimensional physical models can add the sense of touch and immediate 3D manipulations. They are even more intuitive and preparatory than a 3D CT reconstruction alone. There is also the potential for preoperatively practicing procedures on models. Plastic models could be used as a medium for realistic surgical planning, customization of treatment devices, and detailed communication. Models could also be used extensively in educational settings, research, and development.

A potential disadvantage of 3D physical models includes manufacturing costs. They are not immediately available and need several days to prepare. This could be difficult in emergency cases.

DESCRIPTION OF 3D CT IMAGING

The imaging data are derived from routine CT scans of the upper extremity that were obtained for clinical purposes. The best 3D images are created using 0.625- to 1.25-mm slices. The data acquired are fed into medical 3D software (Vitrea 2.0 [Vital Images, Inc, Plymouth, MN, USA] or GE Advantage 4.2 and 4.4 Workstation [General Electric, Milwaukee, WI, USA]), which can create 3D images that can be manipulated for 360° views with the click of a button. Still images are typically saved and stored in the medical record for the surgeon to view, but interested surgeons can go to the radiology area or get a copy of the scan on their computer to manipulate the image into any view (Fig. 1A, B). A series of still images can also be converted into a movie. Most importantly, bones can be subtracted to improve the view of articular surfaces and fracture fragments (see Fig. 1C).

Orthopaedic Hand and Upper Extremity Service, Massachusetts General Hospital, Harvard Medical School, Yawkey Center, Suite 2100, 55 Fruit Street, Boston, MA 02114, USA
* Corresponding author.
E-mail address: dring@partners.org

Hand Clin 26 (2010) 447–453
doi:10.1016/j.hcl.2010.04.007

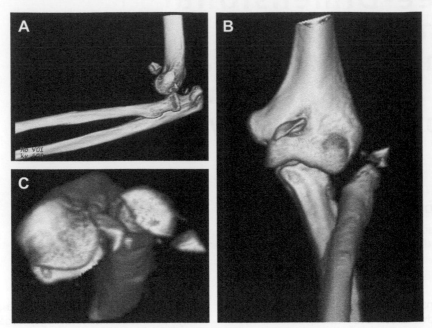

Fig. 1. Three-dimensional lateral (*A*) and anteroposterior (*B*) reconstructions show a terrible triad injury. The articular surface of the radial head and coronoid (*C*) is well visualized when the humerus is removed.

The software to create 3D images is widely available and can be used by surgeons to create their own 3D models. One only needs the Digital Imaging and Communications in Medicine (DICOM) files from the radiologist who performed the CT scan. Many hospitals offer 3D reconstructions, and it is usually as simple as clicking a box on an online form when requesting a CT scan for a patient or paging the radiology technician to let them know the specific need. Radiology staff will produce the 3D reconstructions and upload it to the digital medical record of the corresponding patient.

The cost for a hospital to create its own 3D laboratory depends on the scale and scope of the operation. The cheapest solution would be to use OsiriX,[4] which is provided free of charge under the GNU open-source licensing agreement, and a Macintosh computer (Apple Computers, Cupertino, CA). A more professional single workstation could cost, on the low end, from $20,000 for a Voxar 3D (Voxar, Framingham, MA, USA) to $100,000 to $200,000 for high-end 3D workstations such as a GE Advanced Workstation (General Electric) or Vitrea (Vital Images, Inc, Plymouth, MN, USA). Enterprise-wide 3D systems such as Aquarius Workstation (TeraRecon, San Mateo, CA, USA) or Vitrea Web (Vital Images) can cost $250,000 or more. Maintenance is generally about 15% of the list price. Other expenditures include: 1) 3D technologists (who are generally paid a premium more than that of CT/magnetic

resonance [MR] imaging technologists); 2) cost of training the technologists; 3) developing 3D protocols; 4) supervision; 5) other equipment to acquire, transmit, and store; 6) manipulation and distribution of patient radiological data and imagery over a network (picture archiving and communication systems [PACS]/radiology information systems [RIS]); 7) supplies and overhead. In addition, if the 3D production is done by scanning technologists, they generally do not have the time or expertise to do the more complex work, and it is not efficient to slow down the scan throughput to have a CT/MR technologist spend 30 to 45 minutes to process complex examinations such as head/neck CT angiography. It can be a fairly costly proposition for a large-scale operation, in time, effort, resources, capital, and operating expenses and full-time equivalents (the equivalent of 1 person working full time). It can be done fairly inexpensively by a part-time technician and a low-end 3D system for basic 3D work. Some vendors offer a remote service that gives other hospitals and imaging centers access to a 3D laboratory on a fee-for-service basis, which can be more economical and of better quality than doing the more complex work in-house.

HOW TO CREATE A 3D MODEL

The process of making a 3D CT image starts with retrieving a DICOM file, which is a standard file format for handling, storing, printing, and transmitting information in medical imaging. Retrieval could be done by requesting the radiologist for the required CT image on a CD or by pointing the 3D medical software to the appropriate local network server that stores all the images and searching for the corresponding patient and image. The best-quality 3D models are created with a slice thickness of between 0.62 and 1.25 mm, no underlying cast, and no metal implants. Most 3D medical software allow for searching in the radiology image database as a standard feature. When the requested patient image modality is retrieved into the software, the bone can be manipulated in virtual reality. For example, if the radial head is fractured and one would like to subtract the humeral and ulnar bone, one can select the "free form tool" and erase the humerus and ulna. This manipulation is done by circling and deleting the unwanted bones in each 2D CT slice and then reformatting the 3D image. An isolated view of the radius remains. After this manipulation, images and movies can be created and stored. One can select every requested angle and make a "snapshot" or select the requested rotation and view for a movie. Movies and images can be stored on a local server or on a CD/DVD or added to the patient's digital medical record.

This article explains how to create a 3D model in the free OsiriX[4] software. This program is very straightforward and simple, so it can be used on a Macintosh computer by all orthopedic surgeons.

The program can be downloaded for free online.[5] Unzip and install the program by double clicking the OsiriX Installer icon. The OsiriX navigation uses 3 main windows. The first window is the Database window, where data sets are imported. The second window is the Viewer window, which allows viewing and manipulation of 2D data sets. The third window is the 3D Volume Rendering window, which allows viewing and manipulation of 3D data sets.

The Database window lists the imported data sets and allows one to preview the images. Images are imported by clicking on the Import or CD-ROM icon. The file extension of DICOM files is ".dcm." To view a specific set of images, select the name of the series you would like to open in the patient and study list. Then click on the 2D to 3D viewer button in the toolbar, which opens the Viewer window.

The Viewer window displays data sets from a select series and allows you to manipulate 2D images. The Orientation tool allows the flexibility of changing between axial, coronal, and sagittal views in the preview window. The 3D tool displays data in 3D in a separate window. The 3D viewer is accessed by clicking on the 2D/3D viewer button pull down menu and making a selection. The third window appears once the 3D Surface Rendering selection has been made from the 2D/3D viewer button pull down menu. Preset opacities are available in the Opacity tool. The Manipulate tool moves the object around its center of gravity. The camera position can be changed with the Angle of View tool. The Sculpt 3D Object tool acts as a scissors to cut out specific parts of the 3D model. Click on a bone with the Bone Removal tool, and it will be removed. There are several ways to save and export the created 3D model. The DICOM file tool exports DICOM files. An animated movie can be created with the Fly Thru tool that can be inserted into, for example, PowerPoint (Microsoft, Redmond, WA, USA). A more detailed version of this tutorial with screenshots is available online.[6]

HOW TO CREATE A 3D PHYSICAL MODEL

Three-dimensional physical models are created with the use of a special printer, the Spectrum Z510 3D printer from Z Corporation (Burlington, MA, USA). This printer creates a 3D plastic model, including colors, from a DICOM file (**Fig. 2**). There are also printers to create plaster models.

The process of creating a 3D physical model is usually done by an outside vendor and requires a minimum of 2 days (Medical Modeling Inc, Golden, CO, USA). One should obtain the CT scans at a high spatial resolution, preferably in DICOM format. The suggested technical details for obtaining a proper-quality CT scan for this technique are (1) helical acquisition, (2) field of view to include entire area of interest, (3) gantry tilt of zero degrees, (4) scan spacing with contiguous slices, (5) no reconstruction, (6) slice thickness of 0.75 to 1.25 mm (thickness <3.0 mm is typically acceptable depending on anatomic area), (7) standard algorithm (not bone or detail), and (8) a pitch of 1:1 or 1:1.5. The acquired DICOM file should then be transferred to the vendor, who can usually import image data from most mainstream CT scanners and PACS systems and most storage media.

QUANTITATIVE RESEARCH USING 3D CT AND MODELING TECHNIQUE

The authors' group has developed a technique to quantitatively investigate broken bones with 3D CT.[7] They used the following method: DICOM files were obtained through Vitrea and exported for further processing into Matlab (MATLAB 7.7; The MathWorks, Inc, Natick, MA, USA). With Matlab,

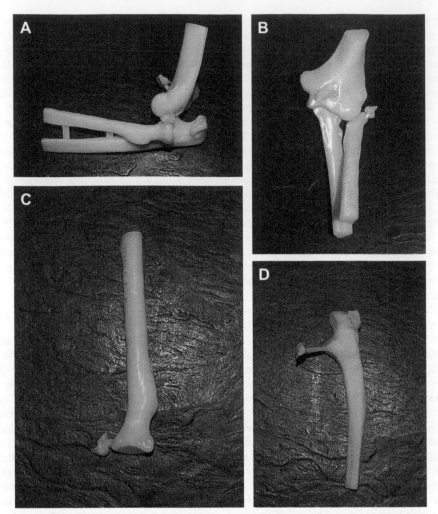

Fig. 2. (*A–D*) Three-dimensional physical models of the same radial head and coronoid fracture.

the CT slides (DICOM) were converted into regular pictures (jpegs) so that they were suitable for further processing.

A special code, written by the Massachusetts General Hospital 3D Imaging Service, aids in this process and identifies higher densities in the CT slides (in essence bony structures). Data describing the relationship between the slides and the higher densities were saved. The created images and the additional created data were then uploaded into Rhinoceros (Rhinoceros 4.0; McNeel North America, Seattle, WA, USA). Rhinoceros is a 3D modeling tool based on NURBS (Non-uniform rational B-spline), a mathematical model commonly used in computer graphics for generating and representing curves and surfaces.

Rhinoceros stacked the images (jpegs) on top of each other, taking their relationship into account.

During the image processing in Matlab, the higher densities (bony structures) are highlighted with points on every CT slide. The actual CT slide is depicted behind the point-wise representation of the bone in the software. The depiction of the CT slide with the points on top of them allows a precise identification of all the bony structures and fragments, even if they were impacted.

The software allows putting in new points on each CT slide, keeping them at the same level as the automatically generated points. After all points were set, we drew lines that then would represent the actual outer border of the bone and so created a wire model (**Fig. 3**A). This wire model was then used to create a polygon mesh (see **Fig. 3**B), which is a collection of vertices, edges, and faces that define the shape of a polyhedral object in 3D computer graphics and solid modeling, consisting of triangles only explicitly representing the surface.

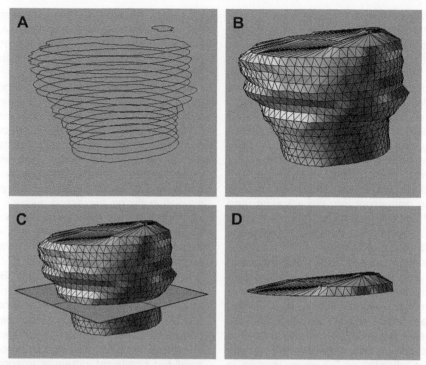

Fig. 3. Creation of the quantitative 3D model from CT data. (*A*) A wire model based on stacking of 2D images. (*B*) The final 3D mesh model of the radial head. (*C*) The cutting plane of the radial head to measure volume. (*D*) The articular surface of the radial head was quantified.

In other words, a hollow 3D model of the outer surface of the bony structures and fragments was generated.

This technique provides the opportunity to learn more about fracture patterns. For example, reconstruction of 3D models can be used to calculate volume and articular surfaces of bones (see **Fig. 3**C, D). When the technique is applied to unfractured bones, one could learn how much volume and articular surface a normal bone has. From this information, mathematical models can be calculated to predict the volume and articular surface that should be present based on specific measurements. This method is of particular value when there is no CT scan of the opposite elbow available. When evaluating the fractured bone, one can calculate the volume and surface area of the fracture fragments and then estimate the percentage fractured and any unaccounted for or "lost" fragments using the mathematical formulas derived from healthy bones. This information is important in research attempting to define, for instance, the number of fragments or the percentage involvement of the proximal articular surface area and may affect the classification and evaluation of these fractures. More detailed and quantitative information concerning the

specific anatomic aspects of bone that could assist the clinician in reconstruction surgery can also be derived from this technique.

One of the disadvantages is that this technique is tedious and time consuming. In addition, there is variability and some subjectivity to the process.

RESULTS IN RESEARCH
3D CT Reconstructions

Harness and colleagues[2] found that the use of 3D CT was superior to 2D imaging alone in characterizing coronal fracture lines and determining the presence of articular comminution and the exact number of articular fragments in distal radius fractures. However, central articular depression was more difficult to assess with 3D imaging alone or in combination with 2D imaging. The investigators concluded that 3D CT improves the reliability and the accuracy of radiological characterization of articular fractures of the distal part of the radius and influences treatment decisions.

Doornberg and colleagues[1] tested the hypothesis that 3D reconstructions of CT scans improve the reliability and accuracy of fracture characterization, classification, and treatment decisions of distal humerus fractures. Five independent observers evaluated 30 consecutive intra-articular fractures of the distal part of the humerus. 3D CT improved the intraobserver and the interobserver reliability of the AO classification system and the Mehne and Matta classification system. 3D CT reconstructions also improved the intraobserver agreement for all fracture characteristics from moderate to substantial agreement. The investigators concluded that 3D reconstructions improve the reliability, but not the accuracy, of fracture classification and characterization.

Lindenhovius and colleagues[8] tested the hypothesis that 3D CT reconstructions improve interobserver agreement on classification and treatment of coronoid fractures when compared with 2D CT. Twenty-nine orthopedic surgeons evaluated 10 coronoid fractures on 2 occasions (first with radiographs and 2D CT and then with radiographs and 3D CT). They concluded that regardless of the imaging modality used, there was fair-to-moderate agreement for most observations. Three-dimensional CT improved interobserver agreement in Regan and Morrey and O'Driscoll classifications. There were trends toward better reliability on 3D reconstruction in recognition of coronoid tip fractures, impacted fragments, and, in surgeons' opinions, the need for something other than screws or plates for operative fixation. They concluded that 3D CT reconstructions improve interobserver agreement with respect to fracture classification when compared with 2D CT.

Brunner and colleagues[3] found that 3D CT reconstructions significantly improved the interobserver reliability to good for the AO/Orthopaedic Trauma Association (OTA) and Neer classifications of proximal humerus fractures. They also found that stereovisualisation of 3D volume–rendered CT datasets significantly improved the intraobserver reliability to good for the AO/OTA classification system and to excellent for the Neer classification system.

3D Physical Models

Bilic and Zdravkovic,[9] found that computerized models[10] facilitated preoperative planning of corrective osteotomy for deformities of the radius. Usui and colleagues[11] and Mahaisavariya and colleagues[12] used similar techniques to plan supracondylar humerus osteotomies in children.

Jupiter and colleagues[13] used a 3D computer-assisted design and manufacturing technology to create solid models of 5 unusually complex, multidirectional malunions of distal radial fractures. Preoperative planning was dramatically enhanced by the ability to perform the surgical procedure on these models, with a model of the uninjured limb used for comparison. All 5 patients had significant malunions, with malrotation in the horizontal plane in 5 and an impacted articular fragment in 2.

Murase and colleagues[14] planned the osteotomy using CT models and executed it using a custom-made osteotomy template. Three-dimensional computer models of the affected and contralateral, normal bones were constructed with data from CT, and a deformity correction was simulated. A custom-made osteotomy template was designed and manufactured to reproduce the preoperative simulation during the actual surgery. When they performed the surgery, the template was placed on the bone surface, the bone was cut through a slit on the template, and deformity was corrected as preoperatively simulated.

In 2009, in an unpublished study, Brouwer and colleagues compared characterization and classification of distal humerus fractures based on 2D CT, 3D CT, and 3D models as compared with intraoperative evaluation as the reference standard. The more sophisticated imaging/models led to small but significant increases in agreement with the reference standard as measured using Kappa statistics.

3D Quantitative Modeling

Our group developed a method to quantitatively analyze fracture fragment morphology on 3D CT images (Q3DCT) in terms of size, shape, volume, and articular surface area. We applied this Q3DCT modeling technique to 46 consecutive adult patients with a fracture of the radial head. The volume and articular surface area of each articular fracture fragment were measured. It was found that partial head fractures (Mason 2) are usually multifragmented and often have fragments that are too small to be repaired according to (admittedly arbitrary) volume criteria and surface area criteria, particularly when the fracture is displaced and unstable. Only 4 of the patients (25%) with whole head fractures (Mason 3) had more than 3 fragments, but 9 (69%) of the fractures with 3 or fewer fragments had irreparable fragments using the same criteria. It was concluded that according to these preliminary data based on modeling using Q3DCT analysis of radial head fracture morphology, partial head fractures are often complex and irreparable, and the criterion of 3 or greater fragments as a threshold for prosthetic replacement of a whole head fracture may not account for all aspects of fracture complexity, including irreparable fragments.

SUMMARY

Previous research has shown that there are multiple advantages of 3D imaging and 3D physical modeling. Three-dimensional reconstructions are more intuitive and lead to improved identification of fracture characteristics, such as fragments, fracture edges, and articular surfaces. This information leads to improved understanding and better preparation of the surgeon. For the patient, it can be of great value in understanding, decision making, and compliance. In addition, 3D reconstructions can have a great impact on education, research, and development. Three-dimensional physical models can add to the advantages of the 3D reconstructions and result in better understanding and surgical preparation, both for the surgeon and the patient.

To our knowledge, measurement of articular surface area and volume has not been attempted in the upper extremity. The promising 3D quantitative analysis technique is important in research attempting to define, for instance, the number of fracture fragments or the percentage involvement of articular surface area. We are using this technique to study fracture fragment size and injury pattern, and the ability to estimate percentage involvement helps make the results more intuitive for clinicians. This may affect the classification and evaluation of fractures. More detailed analysis with these sophisticated techniques may help to influence patient management or implant design.

The technologic advances in imaging of the upper extremity have taken an immense leap in the last decade, so also the amount of research that has been published. Research has shown that 3D reconstructions and physical modeling may outweigh the disadvantages of increased cost, resource usage, and additional time, as both the surgeon and the patient will be benefited significantly.

REFERENCES

1. Doornberg J, Lindenhovius A, Kloen P, et al. Two and three-dimensional computed tomography for the classification and management of distal humeral fractures. Evaluation of reliability and diagnostic accuracy. J Bone Joint Surg Am 2006;88:1795.
2. Harness NG, Ring D, Zurakowski D, et al. The influence of three-dimensional computed tomography reconstructions on the characterization and treatment of distal radial fractures. J Bone Joint Surg Am 2006;88:1315.
3. Brunner A, Honigmann P, Treumann T, et al. The impact of stereo-visualisation of three-dimensional CT datasets on the inter- and intraobserver reliability of the AO/OTA and Neer classifications in the assessment of fractures of the proximal humerus. J Bone Joint Surg Br 2009;91:766.
4. Rosset A, Spadola L, Ratib O. OsiriX: an open-source software for navigating in multidimensional DICOM images. J Digit Imaging 2004;17:205:
5. Available at: http://www.apple.com/downloads/macosx/imaging_3d/osirix.html. Accessed January 6, 2010.
6. Available at: http://www.osirix-viewer.com/Osirix_as_a_Resource.pdf. Accessed January 6, 2010.
7. Guitton TG, van der Werf HJ, Ring D. Quantitative measurements of the volume and surface area of the radial head. J Hand Surg Am 2010;35(3):457–63.
8. Lindenhovius A, Karanicolas PJ, Bhandari M, et al. Interobserver reliability in classification and management of coronoid fractures: two-dimensional vs. three-dimensional computed tomography. J Hand Surg Am 2009;34(9):1640–6.
9. Bilic R, Zdravkovic V. Planning corrective osteotomy of the distal end of the radius. 2. Computer-aided planning and postoperative follow-up. Unfallchirurg 1988;91:575–80.
10. Bilic R, Zdravkovic V, Boljevic Z. Osteotomy for deformity of the radius. Computer-assisted three-dimensional modelling. J Bone Joint Surg Br 1994;76:150–4.
11. Usui M, Ishii S, Miyano S, et al. Three-dimensional corrective osteotomy for treatment of cubitus varus after supracondylar fracture of the humerus in children. J Shoulder Elbow Surg 1995;4:17–22.
12. Mahaisavariya B, Sitthiseripratip K, Oris P, et al. Rapid prototyping model for surgical planning of corrective osteotomy for cubitus varus: report of two cases. Injury Extra 2006;37:176.
13. Jupiter JB, Ruder J, Roth DA. Computer-generated bone models in the planning of osteotomy of multidirectional distal radius malunions. J Hand Surg Am 1992;17:406.
14. Murase T, Oka K, Moritomo H, et al. Three-dimensional corrective osteotomy of malunited fractures of the upper extremity with use of a computer simulation system. J Bone Joint Surg Am 2008;90:2375.

Index

Note: Page numbers of article titles are in **boldface** type.

Hand Clin 26 (2010) 455–458
doi:10.1016/S0749-0712(10)00055-7

hand.theclinics.com

Moving?

Make sure your subscription moves with you!

To notify us of your new address, find your **Clinics Account Number** (located on your mailing label above your name), and contact customer service at:

Email: journalscustomerservice-usa@elsevier.com

800-654-2452 (subscribers in the U.S. & Canada)
314-447-8871 (subscribers outside of the U.S. & Canada)

Fax number: 314-447-8029

Elsevier Health Sciences Division
Subscription Customer Service
3251 Riverport Lane
Maryland Heights, MO 63043

*To ensure uninterrupted delivery of your subscription, please notify us at least 4 weeks in advance of move.

Printed and bound by CPI Group (UK) Ltd, Croydon, CR0 4YY

03/10/2024

01040354-0015